Add Years to Your Life
and Life to Your Years

Add Years to Your Life and Life to Your Years

IRENE GORE

STEIN AND DAY / *Publishers* / New York

First published in the United States of America by Stein and Day/*Publishers* in 1974
Copyright © 1973 by George Allen & Unwin, Ltd.
Library of Congress Catalog Card No. 73-92183
All rights reserved
Printed in the United States of America
Stein and Day/*Publishers*/Scarborough House, Briarcliff Manor, N.Y. 10510
ISBN 0-8128-1685-4

For Olga Youhotsky
whose ageless vitality is a source of joy
and inspiration

Contents

Introduction   *page* 11

PART I: MAN IS SO MUCH MORE THAN A MACHINE
1 The Mechanistic Analogy   15
2 Factors Affecting Longevity   21
3 Causes of Decline in Old Age   27
4 Why Do We Fear Ageing?   33
5 Some Conclusions about Health and Vitality in Old
   Age   39

PART II: SOME ESSENTIAL GENERAL POINTS FOR
          MAINTAINING VITALITY
             (a) THE PHYSICAL COMPONENT OF LIFE
6 Physiological Potential   43
7 The Role of Physical Activity in Physical Well-
   being   46
8 Some Misconceptions about Physical Activity and
   Age   52

PART II (b) THE MENTAL COMPONENT OF LIFE
9 Regarding Life as a Continuum   59
10 Avoiding Some Pitfalls   63

PART III: SOME PRACTICAL SUGGESTIONS FOR
           THE OLDER PERSON ON HOW TO
           MAINTAIN AND IMPROVE PHYSICAL
           AND MENTAL VIGOUR
11 Ageing Well   75
12 Some Guidelines on Positive Health   77

8 /

13 Nutrition 86
14 Dietary Supplements 93
15 Practical Suggestions on Physical Activity 98
16 The Daily Two-Dozen 106
17 Safety Measures 111
18 Mental and Emotional Aspects 116
19 Individual Efforts and the Need for Social Reforms 121
20 Some Glimpses of Longevity 124

Index 131

Add Years to Your Life
and Life to Your Years

Introduction

My motive in writing this book has been to share with older people my hopefulness about ageing.

Research into ageing is still a long way from uncovering the causes and the detailed mechanisms of senescence. But the more we study ageing, the clearer it becomes that decline with the years may be due to many factors other than age. Decline is thus neither universal and uniform, nor inevitable. This being so, one is justified in adopting a positive and optimistic attitude to ageing. This gives one encouragement to take some action towards attaining a healthier and more vigorous long life.

This book attempts to present in some detail the underlying ideas and the evidence upon which such a positive attitude is based. The book also puts forward certain practical suggestions for ways in which we can achieve better health and greater vitality.

Vitality, not youth, is the keyword in this book. Youth is limited in time, which cannot be retrieved. Youth is limited in experience and maturity, which nobody would want to forgo or to jettison. Vitality is not limited in any such way: it can belong to anyone, to any age. It can be cultivated and fostered. Vitality is not a synonym for virility, for sexual desire, or for fertility. Vitality is defined as 'the force of life', 'vital power', 'power of continuing in force'. It embraces physical energy, mental alertness, and enthusiasm in every aspect of living. A man is technically alive as long as his heart continues beating, but nobody would call this living. A man has vitality whether he walks ten miles a day for the sheer pleasure of it, or pores with unflagging interest over a stamp collection. Outward signs of age, such as grey hair or wrinkled skin, do not prevent people from being full of zest and energy, provided they are well.

Since there is no question, and no need, of recapturing youth, this book does not deal with 'rejuvenation'. Monkey glands, magic elixirs and the like are beside the point when there are perfectly *sensible* and simple ways in which we can improve our vigour and vitality. Our minds and bodies can be trained in later years to function better, and will become healthier and more agile – and these are the attributes which are usually regretted as being lost forever with our calendar youth.

At present there is much to be done to dispel the myths and ingrained negative attitudes which shape our ideas about ageing. It is my hope that as more and more elderly people continue to be active and thus preserve their health, the idea that vitality is natural in later years will spread. Ideally, in time, it should become *unremarkable* if people of 80 or 90 ride bicycles or manage a business. Ideally, once adulthood is reached, our age should become irrelevant to our mode of life.

It is a pleasure to acknowledge the help of my husband, Dr Peter Gore, in going over the manuscript. His painstaking attention to detail and constructive suggestions have been invaluable, and have done much to concentrate and clarify the text.

London
April 1972

PART 1

Man is So Much More than a Machine

1
The Mechanistic Analogy

A vital clue to vigour and vitality in later years
Whenever we come across people who are very old in calendar years but who are fit, alert, and vigorous, we tend to wonder how such vitality comes about. Is it through having a knack for preserving strength? Do these people spare themselves every possible mental and physical effort and so conserve their energy? Do they, more than the average person, sit rather than stand, and lie down rather than sit? Have they followed such an energy-sparing mode of life from their youth onwards?

The available evidence shows, perhaps surprisingly to some of us, that such people do not in fact save their energy like a miser hoarding treasure, leaving them with a store of vigour to be squandered in later years. On the contrary, they enjoy a marvellous old age because they have always been active and remain active long past the normal retirement age. Their individual recipes for longevity are legion, but being active and staying active is the common feature in all of them. Keep an eye open for reports of such vigorous people among the famous and the creative, like Pablo Picasso at 90, Pablo Casals at 95, Leopold Stokowski at 90, to name but a few. Not only the famous, but ordinary citizens are reported on from time to time: one who continues full-time gardening at 96; another who regrets having had to retire from cattle-breeding at 87 because of failing eyesight and who comments 'much too early to retire'.

These people have lived a long time, but they are not 'old men'.

Activity indeed holds a vital clue to adding life to our years. The benefit of activity makes complete sense in the light of modern biological thinking, and this will be discussed later.

The mechanistic view of life

When the first steam engines appeared it must have been tempting to draw parallels between living creatures and these self-propelling creations. The parallel seemed relevant indeed with the biological knowledge which existed then, and with the example of people deteriorating physically through years of toil. We still hear, and perhaps use ourselves, stock phrases borrowed from the world of machines when speaking of our bodies: 'wear and tear', 'running down', 'worn out'. This shows that we have some deeply entrenched, and subliminally potent, attitudes towards ageing, coloured by this mechanistic analogy. Let us consider if there is value in this analogy. The basic premise of this parallel is no longer tenable from a biological point of view. The analogy, therefore, is not true. Moreover, it is harmful, as it equates the *use* of the body with its deterioration.

The mechanistic analogy does hold true in one respect. Both our bodies and motor-cars, for example, need an external source of energy (food and fuel, respectively) in order to function. This is where the relevance of the analogy ends. Modern biological work leads to a dynamic, not a mechanistic, view of life. Let us take a look at what this means.

The dynamic view of life

Once a machine is manufactured the materials which go into its making will serve as long as their intrinsic quality and the treatment they receive will allow. Under no imaginable circumstances will the materials be able to renew themselves. With use they will deteriorate. We used to think that this was true also of the human body, but we no longer do.

When radioactive substances became available for biological research after World War II, it became possible for scientists to show quite conclusively that the biochemical components of living organisms exist 'in a state of dynamic equilibrium'. This means that the biochemical components and the resources of our bodies – the materials we are made of and those which we use in order to live – are not laid down once and for all at birth for subsequent use throughout life. These substances are continually synthesized (manufactured) by the body, are used by it, and are synthesized again. This is the process of metabolism, the continual chemical activity which goes on in the body and which keeps us alive. The metabolic processes are fundamental, and they work well only in response to demands made on the body. In other words, if the body *does not use* its resources it stagnates. If it uses its resources, then the body renews itself and its vitality continues. Such is the crucial difference between the constitution of a machine and of a living organism.

There are also differences of functioning. No machine, on any fuel, will gestate, be born, grow, or reproduce. A living organism will do all this, and a great deal more. It can repair itself: we all know how wounds, fractures and other injuries, 'heal themselves'. The body can adapt to a vast range of external conditions and survive. It can mobilize its immunological organization to defend itself against noxious agents. With a machine only an external agency can put right any defect, and a machine cannot adapt itself to conditions much removed from those under which it is meant to perform. If a car loses a wheel, the remaining three cannot do anything to remedy the situation. If a man loses a kidney, the remaining one will grow larger and do the work of both. No matter how much 'training' a family saloon may be subjected to, it will not manage to compete with a racing car in performance. But a man can train himself to perform mental and physical tasks beyond his initial standards. The quality and duration of a machine's performance is thus circumscribed. It will function progressively less well and with long use it will run down, seize up, rust away or otherwise deteriorate. A living organism is much better placed. It has built-in means of self-repair, of self-renewal and of re-establishing its potential. For example, we can recover from an illness or regain the use of an injured limb. We live in a pretty hostile environment, surrounded by all manner of biological threats, yet we manage to keep well most of the time. More and more of us reach old age.

A particularly pernicious corollary to the mechanistic view of life
The likening of the human body to a machine is especially pernicious in connection with ageing. First of all, we know that machines wear out *with use*. If we think of our bodies as machines, we expect them too to wear out with use, i.e. in the course of a long life. Our bodies could wear out, if we toiled incessantly beyond our capacity and in unhealthy conditions. Fortunately, few of us in the developed countries toil like that these days.

Such mechanistic thinking leads us, logically enough, to consider that as we grow older we should 'take it easy', 'slow down', etc., in order to conserve our strength and to prolong our life. This, however, is an unwise course, if we consider what happens to our bodies if they are not used. If a limb is put in plaster, the muscles become wasted and weak. It takes exercise and physiotherapy to return the limb to its normal function. If we are confined to bed, it takes some time for us to regain our strength on getting up. If we undergo surgery, as soon as we are out of the anaesthetic we are encouraged to move our feet, and then to get up as soon as possible, to prevent complications *through activity*. If activity is demonstrably beneficial even when the body has been subjected to acute stress, and its vitality is depleted, then why should we think it wise to curtail our activity as we grow older *just because we are getting older*? In the absence of disease, crushing toil or unbearable mental strain such curtailment will put our health and vigour in jeopardy. It will not preserve our energy and vitality; it will deplete them.

The need for rest

If inactivity is bad for us and activity is good, do we need rest and sleep at all? We obviously do, and the reason for this is fascinating. There is a profound biological difference between inactivity and *rest after effort.* With prolonged inactivity and disuse the various systems of our body become stagnant, they deteriorate and may eventually atrophy. But when we feel tired *after exertion* it is our body clamouring for a period of rest, during which a furious biochemical activity is going on in the organism. Whilst we are active we use up various substances, and this stimulates our metabolism to replenish them and to recharge the organism with energy required for its vital processes. Our tissues and organs are refreshed, flushed out and restored although we are not consciously aware of this. This is the reason why we feel well after a sound sleep following some exertion. The benefits of activity have, therefore, a very sound biochemical basis. This points up further that we cannot equate ourselves with machines. However long we leave a car to 'rest' in the garage after a long journey, it will not of itself be 'restored' in any way, but will be that little bit nearer to becoming decrepit.

Mechanical 'wearing out' versus biochemical malfunction as cause of decline

In the course of our lives some debilitating effects of the stresses and strains of living accumulate. It is easier for us to fend off these effects, or to cope with them, if our organism is functioning properly. This is best achieved if there is a sufficient challenge to the organism. Physical and mental activity provide such physiological challenges. The vitality and well-being of our bodies and minds are interlinked and interdependent. *Mens sana in corpore sano.* The sequence of activity, rest and restoration, and renewed activity can then go full circle. Those of us who keep their vitality and vigour into extreme old age know this instinctively. But too many of us are fearful of wearing ourselves out. This attitude follows a path leading instead towards increasing incapacity, frailty and decline. Our increasingly less active life habits, resulting from more and more technological aids to inactivity, unfortunately foster this lack of exertion. We begin to slow down in our activities in spite of ourselves while we are still young. Even our children abdicate from exertion, as witness the fleets of cars delivering them to school.

Because of all this, it is essential for us to realize just how much our well-being depends on sufficient physical and mental activity. We have the choice to remain, or learn to become, active and thus to grow old in years but fit in body and mind, or to 'save our strength' and to suffer from a protracted decline.

2
Factors Affecting Longevity

Although the *average* life-span of man is at present somewhere near the biblical limit of three-score-and-ten, we all know that some people live less and many live longer than this average age. This is an example of individual variation. It is worthwhile to look at those people who enjoy a long and vigorous life as models of normal, physiological ageing. What factors are involved in making them live longer and better than the average?

Heredity and the biological élite
Scientific inquiry supports the view that heredity is probably the most important factor which determines longevity. To choose one's grandparents wisely has long been a precept for enjoying a long life oneself. If a man's inherited constitution is strong, he will cope with disease, hardship, hunger and other environmental hazards more successfully than a man of weaker constitution. He is likely to survive longer than the average and to keep his vitality to the end. In short, he represents the biological élite. There are such people in any country and in any society. Their constitutions are strong and their instinct for living is unerring. By definition we cannot all be members of an élite, but we can all take a closer look at them, since they are models of that vitality for which we too can strive.

Evidence for the connection between heredity and longevity

A somewhat exotic example of a biological élite was investigated recently by a Russian gerontologist. It was a serious study of communities noted for exceptionally large numbers of documented nonagenarians and centenarians. Such communities are found not only in the splendid climate of the Caucasian mountains, but in the harsher climate of remote regions of Siberia, the Altai mountains and the tundra-like Yakoutia. Environmentally these areas are not favourable to man. Yet unusually large numbers of people living there remain fit and active to a ripe old age. Many of these long-lived inhabitants (even centenarians) do not consider themselves old, and it was confirmed by medical assessments that they were indeed in excellent condition.

It was concluded from these researches that these long-living people are those whose inherited constitution enabled them to survive quite abominable conditions in which their childhood years were spent. They were children about a century ago, when there was enormous infant mortality. There were famines, epidemics, unhygienic living conditions, poverty, lack of any but folk medicine, plus the harshness of nature and climate. In those days there were no means available to tend the weaklings or to nurture them to an age when they could reproduce. For generations only the strongest survived and reproduced, and today's centenarians are their selected offspring. They are indeed members of a biological élite. In this survey most of the people said that their parents had lived to be 80 or 90, which in the mid-nineteenth century was a great age indeed. This exceptionally strong constitution was inherited by the present-day centenarians from their long-lived parents.

The way in which inherited constitution contributed to a long and vigorous life for these people may be illustrated by the following observations on their diets. These people consume vast amounts of animal fats. Diets rich in animal fats are regarded, for people in the developed countries, to be unhealthy. They are believed to contribute to a disease of the arteries, atherosclerosis, a widespread scourge of our times. The incidence of atherosclerosis in these long-lived people was, however, found to be minute. This finding indicates that their inherited constitution enables them to cope with animal fats in quantity without any untoward effects. Their fortunate heredity makes them thrive even under adverse external conditions. Those of us, lacking such heredity, have to take other steps.

Is heredity all-important?
From what I said above it might appear that since we cannot alter our inherited constitution we have no control over our health throughout life, or whether we age well or badly. Fortunately, this is not so. What we are and how we are at any given moment depends on two interacting factors, our heredity and our environment. Our heredity is something we cannot alter, but we can alter our environment so as to give our inherited constitution a better chance.

This point can be illustrated using a horticultural parallel. A plant bred from the best possible stock is allowed to grow for a while and is then deprived of water. The plant will wilt and die, no matter how splendid its inherited constitution, because the environment is no longer able to support its life. On the other hand, a plant bred from moderate, or even inferior, stock may develop into a sturdy specimen if it is provided with the right soil and fertilizer, with the right amount of water and sunlight, in other words with a better environment.

What exactly do I mean by environment in this context? We hear so much these days about the hazards and evils of the pollution of the atmosphere, of rivers and oceans, of towns, of the countryside. All these things do have an important bearing on human life and health. But in the context of this book

I include under environmental conditions not only such differences as living in a grimy city or in the verdant country, in the tropics or beyond the Arctic circle, but also the much more personal criteria of our life habits and our cultural heritage and outlook.

Putting the dread of senility to good use

If we seriously mean to strive for as healthy and active a long life as possible our life habits need to be scrutinized. We all find it enormously difficult to change our habits and our mental outlook, for we are creatures of habit. To achieve this we probably need a real jolt — and fear is usually a very potent agent in this respect. But for fear to be operative, the danger must be sharp and immediate. We would not swallow cyanide, because we fear its immediate and fatal effect. On the other hand the dangers of smoking are not immediate, but insidious, and not 100 per cent fatal — so we continue taking risks. And the infirmities of old age are remote, not fatal, not present in 100 per cent of people over a certain age. In addition, and most importantly, we tend to think that these infirmities are *totally* due to the number of years, and not to the way, a person has lived. We ascribe the infirmities to 'old age' and therefore believe them inevitable. This tendency is regrettable, because it is not based on fact and because it paralyses action. It is not predetermined for us all to decline into a premature and prolonged senility, for there is a great deal we can do to ensure a healthy long life.

I suggested earlier that most of us need a jolt to spur us into revising our views and habits. If we take a good, long look at the worst features of a prolonged senility we shall get just such a jolt. We would, I believe, emerge from such an exercise determined to do everything possible to promote our own fitness and vitality to form a bulwark against dissolution, dependence and decay.

What particular aspects of life need modifying to ensure a healthier and longer active life?
Most of the changes I would advocate are not restrictive in nature. They are to do with expanding, rather than contracting, our range of physical and mental activities throughout life. I do not mean that, from one day to the next, we should all plunge into weight-lifting, or immerse ourselves in the intricacies of nuclear physics. I do mean that we should not get stuck in a groove, or shrink from challenges and novelties, however old we are in years. We should guard against asking too little of ourselves, both physically and mentally, for if we do we shall succeed in subtracting life from our years.

I shall list here (and discuss in more detail later on) some of the factors that can substantially influence the quality of our later life. These factors include diet, exercise, physical and mental challenges, a sufficient variety of impressions and contacts with the world, a reasonable philosophy of life, an expectation of well-being. How far we benefit from these factors entirely depends on our will and our choice. The benefits of expanding rather than contracting our involvement with life rest on the ideas I mentioned in Chapter 1. An expansionist attitude makes sense because there is growing evidence that people retain their *potential* vitality even in extreme old age. One wonders more and more how many elderly people decline not because they run out of potential, but because their potential is not sufficiently called into play.

It is not easy to explain the precise meaning of 'potential'. I shall attempt to do so in Chapter 6, but for the moment it may be helpful to illustrate the presence of potential in elderly persons by describing two rather extreme cases. Both concern elderly ladies, who appeared to be senile old women, and who could have been written off as victims of old age. Fortunately, they were properly examined. One, aged 70, was found to be very anaemic and depressed, and the other, aged 80, was malnourished and suffered from severe vitamin B deficiency. Both responded dramatically to treatment and became their former *selves*. Their potential vitality was realized through the medication they needed. They were no longer 'senile old women'. These were not miracles but the response of the body's potential to bio-chemical interference.

This brings me to a habit many of us have and which needs questioning and changing. To expect to feel less than well as we grow older is a habit inimical to successful ageing. It is normal to feel well; if we feel 'under the weather' we should seek out the cause and attend to it, instead of brushing it off as 'just old age creeping up'. With such a *laissez-faire* attitude it will not be old age, but a collection of infirmities and disabilities which will creep up on us.

Perhaps it is psychologically unfortunate that in our culture no stigma is attached to physical ailments and lack of fitness. On the contrary, the ailing receive greater care and attention. If an ailment is not too taxing, there is no social pressure on us to attend to it. In some cases perhaps we even tend to 'enjoy poor health', as the saying goes. There is no harm in 'enjoying' poor health occasionally; but as a way of life it is a thoroughly unsatisfactory road into old age.

If we wish to remain active and independent in our calender old age, then we have to work at it. This means looking sensibly after our health, and questioning, and adapting some of our attitudes, habits and activities. It may be difficult, it may seem a nuisance, but if it helps us to remain involved in the world around us, to retain our vitality, and to keep our independence, then it is well worth it.

3
Causes of Decline in Old Age

Physical decline

We tend to assume that the main reason for a decline in vitality is the passage of time. In fact other factors may be responsible for such symptoms as we observe. This confusion is understandable because the position is very complex, as I shall try to illustrate.

There is a widely-held notion that old age is automatically accompanied by infirmities and disabilities. When we see frail, listless, pale elderly people most likely we think that the root cause of their state is their age. 'They are not getting any younger.' A more worrying aspect of the situation is that the elderly people themselves will most likely judge their situation similarly. They will therefore tolerate their lack of energy and vitality as an inevitable accompaniment of their ageing. In so doing they will progressively decline. It is necessary to realize that there may be many other reasons for the observed symptoms. Heredity may be responsible for a weak constitution. These people may have a long and unfortunate medical history. Their nutritional status may be poor – they may be anaemic or have a vitamin deficiency. They may be depressed because of a bereavement, or because of financial worries; they may be bored or lonely. These are all real enough problems, but they are not rooted in the relentless and irreversible passage of time. At least an attempt can be made to resolve them. Health and vitality could then improve and the decline be arrested even though time itself marches on. It pays to check whether it is in fact the abuse, misuse or disuse of our bodies which brings about decline, and to take remedial measures.

When large numbers of reasonably fit elderly persons were screened at special clinics in London and Glasgow, astonishing numbers of pathological conditions were uncovered. If these had gone undiscovered the elderly people would have continued ascribing their infirmities to their old age.

I think we tend too often to look at *pathological* old age and to think of it as *physiological* (or normal) old age. Investigations on very long-lived people, including centenarians, such as are being carried out at the Institute of Gerontology in Kiev, should provide a model of what normal old age is really like.

It rests with us as individuals to take the initial step in safeguarding ourselves as we grow older. A doctor can fortunately carry out various tests and assessments on an elderly person and diagnose whether there is any medical cause for any untoward symptoms. A crucial point about any attempt to prevent decline is this: we must be aware that to be old does not necessarily mean to be weak or ill. If we do feel weak, or listless, or unwell, then we should seek medical advice.

Mental Decline
It is indeed easy to mistake the causes of a decline in mental alertness and flexibility which we observe in some older people. We see them become increasingly apathetic and finding it progressively more difficult to muster their mental resources or to grapple with new ideas. We tend to regard these changes as inevitable, as being due to the passing of the years, and we are afraid of what the future may hold for us. But if these changes are not necessarily due to age, then what other reasons may there be? Disease, such as cerebral atherosclerosis, can lead to eventual mental deterioration. But this is not ageing. It is a pathological

condition. In the absence of disease mental decline may be simply due to a gradual diminution of mental exercise. This may be almost imperceptible over the years, and dictated not by age but by the circumstances of life. In our middle years many of us are preoccupied with a comparatively narrow range of pursuits: we attend to our careers or to our families. We lack the time or the opportunity to widen our horizons or to refresh our impressions and our thoughts. In later years we then have little to fall back on, and our mental input diminishes still further. If input diminishes, so does our response. Apathy and increasing difficulty in mustering our mental resources will be the eventual result. For just as muscles waste through inactivity, so do minds become sluggish and inert without fresh challenges. This is the situation which we fear, but one we can do much to forestall.

We can help to preserve and extend our mental vitality by keeping in touch with contemporary trends and events. By drawing on the works of past generations we can derive delight and stimulation. With modern library facilities, with radio, television and records all these things are so easily available, and those of us who are not creative by nature can expand and enrich our lives through the creations of others.

To be creative, in however limited a way, is of course a great boon, and a veritable fountainhead of vitality. We all know what tremendous satisfaction people get out of gardening, or out of handicrafts. This is true at all ages: one only has to think of how much importance is attached, and rightly so, to creative activities in schools. Many elderly people get a new lease of life when they try their hand at painting or some other art or craft. Our mental state has a direct physiological bearing on our well-being. This is not merely a 'mind over body' pet theory. The more biologists learn about the way we function, in biochemical terms, the more it is realized that 'mind' and 'body' are interdependent. It is a circular situation: an alert mind helps the body to keep its vigour; an active body helps the mind to function properly.

Research into ageing
How easy is it for a scientist studying the ageing process to
discern which changes in an organism are due directly to the
passage of time? It is not easy at all. A living organism is an
enormously complex system, and so to isolate one criterion, such
as age, in any scientific study is very difficult indeed. However,
the more work is done on ageing, and the more critically we
assess the evidence, the clearer it becomes that much of the
decline observed may in fact be due to other causes than age
itself. This development offers hope. We cannot alter the passage
of time, but we can manipulate other conditions of life and thus
prevent or ameliorate the miseries often associated with old age.
At this point it may be of interest to take a look at the way
research into ageing is designed.

How do scientists study age phenomena?
Many of our ideas on how people (or animals in laboratory
experiments) change with age stem from so-called cross-
sectional studies. Tests (e.g. physiological, biochemical, physical,
psychological) are carried out on groups of people of one age
and the results are compared with those obtained from similar
tests on groups of people of another age. For results to be
meaningful and as representative of a general situation as possible
the groups being compared should comprise large numbers of
individuals. After all, even if a group of people is matched for
age and sex each individual will differ in many respects from the
others. Cross-sectional studies are therefore only an approximate
method of finding out something about any particular age group.
They can only provide approximate guidelines for what is
regarded as normal (the 'norm') for that age. The more refined
the methods employed in a study, the more exceptions emerge,
making it very difficult to generalize.

Much more interesting are the so-called longitudinal studies.

Here the same individuals are investigated at intervals of time. In other words we get a picture of how an individual (and not a composite representative of an age group) changes in his test score over the years. Even so in these studies we are observing the effects due only to the passage of time, only if we take very elaborate precautions to sift off as many of the other factors as possible. The practical difficulties of such longitudinal studies are, therefore, great. They are of necessity extremely long-term, and need a great deal of cooperation and follow-up work. The numbers involved must be sufficient to enable us to draw valid general conclusions about ageing.

In cross-sectional studies we try to assess how an individual of a particular age might score, judging by the data obtained from a group of people of that age. In longitudinal studies we learn a great deal about the changes that occur in individuals as they grow older.

The choice before us
An author I met recently put forward an intriguing idea. He suggested that perhaps, for the first time in human history, we have an actual choice of how we shall age. In former times the conditions of life were healthier in so far as people were forced to be more active physically than we are, their food was more natural, there was less industrial pollution. On the other hand, many toiled beyond their strength. There were epidemics, insufficient food, lack of hygiene, lack of medical help. All these factors prevented the majority of people from living on into old age. These various threats to our health and longevity are no longer prevalent, but others rear their heads. We have to recognize them and to combat them. These threats are primarily those of over-nutrition and under-exertion. If we drift on, making our daily life more and more automated, our legs and muscles will become redundant; if we rely more and more on a predigested mental diet, our minds will not thrive. If we allow ourselves to be carried

unthinkingly along the stream of modern life it will bring us to physical and mental malfunctioning and decline long before we reach a ripe old age. That is one way we may elect to take. The other way we may choose is to take advantage of all the benefits of modern civilization, and to try to avoid its disadvantages. We can use what modern knowledge has to offer us on nutrition, exercise, health, medicine, hygiene, mental health, emotional satisfaction. We can use modern facilities for being in contact with the world around us, and for travel and communication. At the same time we should recognize the obverse side of the modern way of life, and to modify it in a personal context so as to provide ourselves with the maximum possible physical and mental training. We can thus have a better chance of health and vitality in old age.

To have such a choice before us is a privilege. To make the choice may not be easy, it may be an effort to regulate our life rather than to drift along. But as more and more of us live longer lives we as individuals have to give thought to making the extra years a boon, and not a burden to ourselves.

4
Why Do We Fear Ageing?

The image of old age

Our times are very much an era of the 'image'. The word is rather interesting, if we analyse it. It has connotations of being a façade; of presenting a view of the subject but not necessarily the whole of it; even, in some cases, of hiding or falsifying its reality. Since our present-day culture does not seem to lay much store by experience and since it does not venerate our elders, our 'image' of old age is largely negative. Most people do not look forward to growing old, because they fear becoming frail, helpless and dependent. Naturally such prospects are frightening. But should they loom so large in our view of old age?

It seems to me that a certain amount of understandable ignorance plays a part in creating such a pessimistic attitude to old age. Most of us know of elderly people who are frail, helpless or dependent. What we do not always appreciate is that most likely they are also not well. I dealt with this crucial point in Chapter 3. Ill health is a handicap at any age. In calendar old age a great deal of minor ill health need never be tolerated if we do not accept it as 'natural' once we are 'past our prime'. This phrase is itself an example of how a period of life is arbitrarily assumed to be the peak period of the life-span. There are people who are listless and apathetic at 20; others who are full of energy and vitality at 50; others still who are vigorous and alert at 80. At any age ill health or dormant conditions which could, if neglected, lead to ill health should be prevented or treated. If we know that good health can be enjoyed even in extreme old age, then the fear of becoming *inevitably* helpless and frail will recede.

Apart from the reproductive aspect chronological age is not so important after we reach adulthood. In a sense our notion of when 'old age' begins has altered most remarkably over the last half-century or so. We have only to think of a Victorian lady of about 50 and her counterpart today, to realize how far we have pushed the frontier of 'old age'. The Victorian woman and the modern woman at 50 look, act, think and live in ways which make them appear to belong to different generations. This difference cannot be due to the process of biological evolution, since a half-century is in evolutionary terms infinitesimal. On the other hand physical, mental and social conditions of life have changed radically in this half-century. These days most people of about 50 live far more actively and youthfully than did their Victorian counterparts. I would suggest that conditions which now prevail allow people of today in some ways to retain their vigour. They live according to their physiological rather than calendar age, and so are not prematurely old, rigid and sedate. It is my contention that this process of pushing the frontiers of 'old age' further and further away is continuing. It can be accelerated through our growing knowledge of how we function and through giving some thought to the individual and the social aspects of ageing.

The role of the mass media in forming our image of old age
It is regrettable that the press, radio and television tend too often to present old age in an unhappily one-sided way. I believe that they do this from the best of motives. They are trying to awaken the conscience of society to the plight of those elderly people who need help, who are lonely, destitute, ill, bed-ridden, institutionalized, and so on. I am sure the media achieve some response and some amelioration of the situation for some of these people. But at the same time they do a disservice to most of

us, young and old, by thus concentrating on the negative aspects of 'old age'. Such emphasis makes the problem appear to be overwhelmingly difficult and sad; we respond by feeling pity, guilt and fear – all negative emotions – which in fact often paralyse action.

I know of course that such unfortunate, elderly people do exist, and they deserve all possible care and help and attention. But they are not representative of what biological ageing has in store for *everyone*. In a sense, if every report on children dealt with spastic children, autistic children, battered babies, orphans, mentally retarded children, mongols, thalidomide victims, and deaf and dumb children, we would be tempted to assume that these reports represented a picture of childhood at the present time. But we do not generalize from these special cases to the majority of our children. Whatever special action needs to be taken to help these particular groups of children, it does not follow that there is no need to plan and improve the life and education of quite normal children, to give the majority a better chance in life. Similarly, whilst those elderly folk who are in unfortunate circumstances should, without any doubt at all, be helped and sustained, the welfare of the majority of the ageing also needs some thought. This majority will age better given more knowledge and the courage to face the passage of time with equanimity. A truer and more positive image of 'old age' would help a good deal in this context.

Some examples of a more positive approach in the mass media
Having said some harsh things about the mass media, I must in fairness say that, by keeping a sharp lookout for items to do with ageing, one can glean some positive reports from time to time. There was, for instance, the excellent recent series of TV programmes 'Seventy plus', under the chairmanship of Professor Ferguson Anderson, which dealt with many problems of the elderly in a sensible, positive, informative and optimistic way.

Some of the people who appeared on this programme were a joy to watch and to hear. For instance, the members of a cycling club, with members aged 70 and upwards, who were full of life and vigour; or the ladies who spoke with animation and delight of a new world opening before them since they took up painting. A few months ago there was a splendid gentleman approaching his 100th birthday, who spoke in a clear strong voice about having driven a combine-harvester at 95, and ridden a horse at 99. There was a lady of 85 interviewed on a Welsh beach in the middle of winter. She has a swim every day of the year. She is straight and agile, with lively eyes. When asked why she was still swimming at her age, she replied that *she had never seen any reason for giving it up, she enjoyed it and it made her feel well*. She had had illnesses in the course of her life, but that had not deterred her from leading an active life.

The newspapers report from time to time various stories about people of astonishing energy and verve in their 80s and 90s. Sir Barnes Wallis has no intention of giving up his aeronautical inventions and designs although he is now 84. Field Marshal Sir Claude Auchinleck, who is 87, is photographed at a ceremony at Sandhurst, a splendid figure of a man. A gentleman of 85 is reported to be active in a gravel business he owns, farming 400 acres of land, and training race horses. Britain's 'oldest working man', 96, does a full week's gardening job. All this makes splendid reading. Quite obviously the papers do not scour the land for this information, but just publish the bits that come up from time to time. If they really wanted to make a feature of presenting fit, active, contented people, who are chronologically old but *who hardly realize how old they are*, I am sure they would find a great number of them.

There is a particular reason why I wish the mass media did more towards projecting a positive image of ageing. To know of active and vigorous elderly people among our own population would mean more to us than to read about the amazingly long-lived and healthy tribes (such as the Hunzas) in the Himalayas, or about people in Kazakhstan or Yakoutia, who live under cultural and climatic conditions very different from ours. It would also mean more to us than to know about the undiminished greatness in old age of such creators as Verdi (who composed *Falstaff* in his 80s) or Titian (carried off by the plague, aged 99) in the past, or Artur Rubinstein, or Sir Adrian Boult, both splendid performing musicians in their 80s, in our own day. These are men of great gifts, and we may feel that what happens to them does not in the least apply to us. It is of course a tremendous boon to have such gifts, for with them one can go on doing that which one does superbly well. But, with all their gifts, these people also continue to strive for perfection; they do not rest on their laurels or shun challenges because 'they are not getting any younger'. And in this there is a hint for all of us. However modestly gifted we may be, to foster our vitality it is important not to shrink from challenges, however modest, trivial, or indeed formidable they may be.

Challenges as a source of vitality
Challenges, if met, bring confidence and confidence makes it easier to meet fresh challenges. I use the word 'meet' advisedly: it does not necessarily presuppose success, but a willingness to have a go. Such willingness lies on the circular path, starting from a spark of vitality which leads to action, and this in its turn promotes further vitality. It often seems to me that people repeat such phrases as 'it becomes more difficult to learn new things as you grow older, doesn't it?' more as an excuse for not bothering than as an observation of fact. It may be more difficult to *concentrate* on learning something new for various reasons: we may be distracted by other duties or cares; we may lack confidence; or we may have simply got out of the habit of tackling anything new. Research is questioning more and more the preconception that the intrinsic ability to learn declines markedly with age

unblemished by disease. If we go on being receptive to new things, we shall enrich our lives and gain vitality without bothering our heads about whether it is more difficult to absorb new things, or not.

An antidote to the fear of old age

The fears we have about old age are real and justifiable only so long as the negative aspects of ageing are disproportionately emphasized in so much of what is presented to us. These fears are real so long as we ascribe the bad effects of disease or of our life-habits to the passage of time. Our life-habits are dictated sometimes by our circumstances, sometimes by our cultural stereotypes, sometimes by ignorance or indolence, or a combination of these. This imposes limitations on our bodies, our senses and our minds. These factors and not age itself are responsible for most of the decline we fear. This being so, the antidote to our fears is to seek out the positive in ageing, to realize that we have physical and mental *potential* which can endow us with vitality no matter how old we grow. We *grow* old. A splendid phrase, this, if we stop to think about it. To grow is to increase, to enlarge and to progress; it negates the warping notion that to age is to contract, to limit and to impoverish our life.

5

Some Conclusions about Health and Vitality in Old Age

The main purpose of the first part of this book has been to show that it is *possible* to enjoy health and vitality even in extreme old age. To do so we need not become health-obsessed hypochondriacs. We do need to accept that ill health, weakness and disability are not *inevitable* accompaniments of old age. The corollary follows that any aches or pains or discomforts, if they are more than fleeting, should be seen to and not ignored. We should not be content to put up with them simply because 'we are not getting any younger'. Taking reasonable care is not fussing over our health, but a sensible way of preventing further disabilities or chronic ill health. It is a way of preserving our independence.

Good health is a solid basis for vitality but it is not the only one. To foster vitality we need to present our bodies and our minds with sufficient challenges and to have an expansionist attitude to life rather than an isolationist one. We know from experience that a person restricted physically and mentally over a period of time deteriorates both in body and mind. This deterioration can be dramatic, if for instance a man spends several months by himself in a cave. The decline can also be insidious, our vitality being eroded over the years if we progressively limit ourselves in our physical and mental activities. As animal organisms we need movement for our bodies to function properly. We are also thinking creatures who need outside stimuli for our minds to work on. Some people are blessed with vitality by nature, and their example serves as a model of normal ageing. They do not go through life cellophane-wrapped against all adverse influences. They are so biologically constituted that their organisms are able to *cope* better than the average with adverse factors; they are better equipped for adaptation to unfavourable circumstances and for regulation of any imbalances; their capacity for self-repair and self-renewal is greater. All this makes them members of a biological élite. But those of us who are not so fortunately endowed do need to take some thought about the best ways of fostering our vitality and thus to safeguard our old age from premature decline.

If we think of ourselves as machines, then we are bound to take a pessimistic view of ageing. For machines wear out, become useless and end up on the scrap heap.

If we think of ourselves as living organisms which thrive on action and reaction, on challenge and response, we are justified in taking an optimistic view of ageing. We are capable of self-repair, of a recharging of energy and a restocking of metabolic requirements. It is largely up to us to ensure that we age well, by creating a favourable personal environment for ourselves. It is easier for us to see how this can be achieved in a commonsense way, if we understand better how we function.

The remainder of the book is concerned with this aspect.

PART II

Some Essential General Points for
Maintaining Vitality

(a) The physical component of life

6
Physiological Potential

Part II of this book is concerned with further aspects of fostering physical and mental vitality throughout life.

What is potential

Physiological potential can be regarded as those latent resources of our organism, which are capable of coming into action when called upon. This potential is not a *store* of energy, but the *capacity* to supply energy.

When is potential present?

For a healthy view of ageing it is fundamental to appreciate that physiological potential exists throughout life. Our potential enables us to respond to physiological challenges, to repair injuries and damage, to improve our performance and to increase our vigour through training, by calling our innate resources into play.

In most people's minds the word and concept of 'potential' is applicable only to youth. It is very easy to demonstrate the presence of physiological potential in children. They quite obviously grow taller, stronger, more skilled; they learn new things at school and their mental horizons expand. In children the rate of expansion is very fast; so it is easy to observe their potential being realized. It is not so easy to demonstrate the presence of potential in adults. Once we have matured, our potential goes underground, as it were. In fact it continues to regulate and govern all our functions but we are not specifically aware of it. However, it becomes easy to demonstrate our potential in situations of crisis, when it emerges to deal with any given disturbance. If, for example, an adult falls ill or is injured he can recover, sometimes with medical help, sometimes even without it, because his physiological potential responds to the challenge and his body is restored to its normal state.

The question arises whether physiological potential exists also in old age. As in younger adults, so in the elderly physiological potential operates subtly. We can let it lie dormant or call it into play. There may be more or less potential according to our heredity. Our mode of life may, or may not, allow its maximum development. But it is always there. To demonstrate the presence of potential in elderly people we again have to turn to situations of crisis. Doctors in geriatric practice constantly rely on this potential in their work. They successfully treat illnesses or perform surgical operations, and their patients, however old they are, recover. If it were a medical fact that once a certain age is reached, there is no more physiological potential to call upon, then doctors would not attempt any treatment, but could only make their patients above this given age as comfortable as possible. But if an old lady breaks her leg she is not left to lie in bed till the end of her days. She is operated upon if necessary, her bones are set and they *knit*. Her physiological potential for self-repair has been realized. She is then given physiotherapy and exercises so that her muscles and tendons realize their potential for resuming normal functioning. The patient eventually becomes mobile again and returns to independence. In cases of mental disturbance there is also good response when the treatment is based on the assumption that potential for improvement exists.

In normal, non-crisis, situations the way elderly persons can convince themselves that they have potential is by extending their efforts. They should try, gently and gradually, to push themselves to do a little more than they have been doing. The particular type of activity is unimportant: it may be getting up from the chair, or walking, or climbing stairs, or gardening. This approach constitutes training – making our potential manifest. It is a very heartening fact that studies comparing elderly and young people have shown that training produces in the two groups a similar *relative increase* in muscular strength and working capacity.

We shall benefit greatly if the idea that physiological potential exists throughout life takes root in our minds, and leads to sensible action. Using our potential leads to successful living and successful ageing. Essentially it forms the foundation for improving the quality of our life, be it in childhood, adulthood, maturity or in calendar old age. We need not fear physical or mental activity of sensible proportions, however old we are, but to welcome it. It is inactivity which we should fear.

7
The Role of Physical Activity in Physical Well-being

The relation between physical activity and the functioning of the body
Physical activity is said to be essential for physical well-being. But why should exercising a few muscles in our legs or in our arms be so important? If all this exercise could achieve would be stronger arms or bulging leg muscles, its importance would indeed be limited. This situation would exist if our bodies were so constructed that each part functioned independently of the others. In fact, nothing could be further from the truth. The whole wonder of a living organism is the way its separate parts and systems and functions are integrated with one another. They are interdependent and exert a profound influence one upon the other. Most biological processes are cyclical, and the cycles are linked, so that events in one engage those in another. There is an exchange of 'signals', be they chemical or electrical. The body's functions are regulated by 'feedback', activation, inhibition, coordination, and so on. All these things act in harmony and are balanced when the organism is working properly. The 'organism' is our physical body, which is constructed and which functions in the most refined, complex and precise manner. It is quite unsurpassed even by the most admired technological inventions and processes devised by man. 'We' are this physical body (organism) plus our characteristics of psyche and personality.

We use the facilities of our organism, without giving much thought to it, unaware of all the tremendous activity which goes on in it all the time. This unawareness is useful but up to a point only. Since we have such splendid physiological equipment we should not take it for granted entirely. We should take some care to provide it with the best conditions under which it can attain maximal expression of its capacity. The processes within the organism are interdependent, but they are also dependent on the conditions we provide for them in our way of life. Our mode of life can influence profoundly the functioning of our organism – for good or ill.

It is in this context that the real importance of physical activity becomes intelligible. Movement is an integral part of being alive and therefore physical activity is the natural, physiological stimulus to which the whole organism responds positively. Exercise does not affect only the size and strength of our muscles. It uses them as trigger points for activating our metabolism as a whole.

Many studies on patients have demonstrated that exercise has beneficial effects on a variety of disturbances, e.g. impaired circulation, respiration, hormonal balance, joint mobility, nervous and muscular coordination, blood chemistry, and digestion. Equally, in healthy people habitual adequate physical activity, which is neither excessive nor minimal, helps to keep systems unimpaired and to continue functioning properly.

Let us examine next how physical activity can produce such profound effects on the various systems of our bodies.

Perhaps the most obvious effect is that stronger muscles provide better support for the skeleton. This prevents damage to the joints and to the spine, which would otherwise have to bear excessive weights. Mobility further protects the skeleton by preventing loss of calcium from the bone-tissue; such loss would result in a thinning and weakening of the bones.

The performance of the cardio-vascular system is improved by exercise. The heart pumps blood through the network of blood vessels throughout the body. When we use our legs in walking, the squeezing action of the leg muscles helps to return the blood from the leg veins to the heart, and it has been estimated that this reduces the load on the heart by 30 per cent. Physical activity helps blood circulation in another way, through opening a network of capillaries (small blood vessels), which remain largely closed (non-functioning) when a person is habitually inactive. Some of the work-load on the large, vital blood vessels is taken off by this collateral circulation, and the tissues are provided with a more effective blood supply. This means that they receive adequate nutriments and oxygen from the blood, and return to the blood the accumulated waste-products. Since our respiration is enhanced by activity the gas exchange in the lungs becomes more effective: we breathe in more air (and therefore more oxygen) and dispose of more of the waste carbon dioxide and water vapour in the air we breathe out.

Exercise raises our metabolic rate, which means that the turnover of foodstuffs in our body is more rapid, and more energy becomes available. Our appetite improves, and the secretion of digestive juices is stimulated. The excretory organs of the body, i.e. kidneys bowels and skin, are activated.

Exercise also has a profound influence on our nervous system. Each voluntary muscular movement we make, be it playing the piano, or walking, or making beds, or wagging our ears, entails a complex and coordinated series of signals and responses between the muscles, the nerves and the brain. The more we make use of these 'pathways', the better 'tuned' our bodies will become. The brain also needs outside stimuli for a very important function, namely our orientation in space. If we are immobile and are denied visual, auditory and tactile experiences, we lose our 'body image' (our instinctive appreciation of our dimensions) and the sense of our configuration in space (whether we are situated the right way up).

Adverse biological reaction to inadequate physical activity in old age
Research has shown that, physiologically, older organisms react
more adversely to inadequate physical activity than do younger
ones. Thus, in laboratory experiments on rats it has been demonstrated that young rats who were forced to remain inactive lived,
on average, for 82 days after the start of mobility restriction.
Young rats who were free to move about normally lived 530 days
from the same date. Old rats subjected similarly to restricted
mobility lived only 30 days from the beginning of the experiment.
Another experiment was designed to ascertain whether it was immobility, i.e. disuse of muscles and consequent loss of the physiological stimulation of the organism, or some other factor, which
produced such an adverse reaction. Groups of rats were kept under
identical conditions in every respect, except that one group was
kept completely immobile, another group was allowed into
spacious cages for half an hour a day, and animals in another
group were made to support themselves for half an hour a day
on vertical posts through their own muscular efforts. At the end
of the three weeks of experiment, 40 per cent of the immobile
rats had died, but only 6 per cent died of those rats which had
been allowed the daily half-hour exercise period. It is remarkable
that even a very limited amount of activity can be so beneficial.
These are thought-provoking findings, for in this context
experiments on animals can serve to indicate what might happen
also with human beings.

Whilst older people do not need to exercise especially hard,
their bodies do need, and do benefit from, an active mode of life.
Why their need for the physiological stimulus of activity is
greater than that of younger people is not entirely clear at present. It may be due to their having allowed themselves, in the
course of a long life, to become 'out of condition'. It may also,
at least in part, be due to various pathological changes in their
organism resulting from injuries or illnesses sustained by it over

a long life. To know the precise *reason* for this greater need for physical activity is however not especially important for us. What is important is to realize that this need exists. We know that children benefit from being active. We are increasingly aware that the middle-aged benefit from exercise. We may not be sufficiently aware, as yet, that the chronologically elderly may be the ones who benefit most from being sufficiently active. Given reasonable health, an active life does not become inimical to health at any age. As we become less active, our muscles provide less stimulation for the rest of the organism, and the longer the body lacks this the more 'out of condition' it will become. Sluggishness, weakness, difficulties in coordination, malfunction and degenerative troubles of circulation and mobility may eventually develop. Some would call this picture 'Old Age'; but it is not produced by the passage of *time*.

Practical hazards of diminishing activity
The hazards of restricted mobility and restricted activity for the ageing are very real indeed. We know that sometimes we feel very tired at the end of a day when we had exerted ourselves physically only very little. We then go to bed early. We wake up, potter around, feel tired, have a sleep after lunch and again feel tired by the evening. But then sleep cannot bring proper refreshment after an inactive day. For sleep after inactivity is not equivalent to rest after exertion. It is the exertion which consumes some of our resources and nudges the body to rest up, allowing the biochemical restocking of these resources and the provision of extra potential energy for future use. In this case we do feel 'rested' after a good sleep. It is unfortunate that we cannot readily distinguish between the sensation of tiredness after exertion and the sensation of tiredness through lack of activity. The situation I have just pictured could describe a typical day in the life of many elderly people, and would be regarded as normal

by them. It is, however, such a quiet life which is a hazard for health and independence.

A direct consequence of inadequate movement is the eventual restriction of mobility of limbs and joints which is likely to occur. Mobility is more important than any other factor for ensuring independence in our daily lives. A vicious circle is set up: diminished ability to move → diminished activity → diminished vitality → diminished impetus to move, and so on. Physical sluggishness leads to circulatory and joint troubles, to a lowered resistance to infection, to slower recovery from any illness or injury, and to disability. In other words, it leads to pathological old age and its attendant infirmities. This is the situation which we rightly fear, but which we can do much to avoid.

8

Some Misconceptions about Physical Activity and Age

Some physiological processes occur at fairly specific ages. Thus, milk teeth erupt in infancy, and permanent teeth are usually complete before puberty. Most people reach puberty sometime between the ages of 12 and 15. Most women reach the menopause between 40 and 50. There is no clear correlation, however, between the capacity for physical activity and age. Some children are slow and sluggish; young people are not all athletic; some middle-aged people are sedentary and flabby, others are mobile and wiry; some elderly people sit in a chair all day, whilst some of their contemporaries dig in the garden or go for long walks. Our activity is much more closely related to our state of health, to our life-habits and to our personal preferences, than to age as such. Children can spend many hours playing with a ball. Elderly people are not likely to do this, because they have not the interest in this pastime; but this does not mean that they are *incapable* of this activity.

There is no natural law against continuing to be physically active throughout life. And yet many of us *assume* that we become less and less capable of activity with the passage of time, without necessarily putting this assumption to the test. We demand less of ourselves, and we do not keep up former activities and skills. We certainly do not strive to develop new ones. In this way we gradually lower our standards, being content with decreasing achievement. In so doing we jeopardize our health and vitality and our chances of a rewarding and independent long life. In the absence of disease or disability such an assumption of a decreasing capacity is not justified. Our bodies only function properly when sufficient, i.e. neither overwhelming nor minimal, demands are made on them. We are not justified in

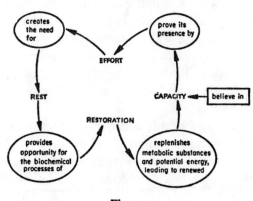

Figure 1

assuming that we have a dwindling store of strength and energy, which needs to be conserved. At any moment of our life we subconsciously feel that the particular way we live, and the amount of activity we have, are those natural to us and to our situation. They may be *natural*, but they are not necessarily *optimal*. This means that we may be functioning adequately enough, but not nearly as well as we might, if we gently pushed ourselves a little. Those elderly people who keep their vitality extend themselves instinctively, and so maintain the cycle (see Figure 1) of effort, rest, restoration, and capacity for more effort. Such people feel no decrease in capacity, and do not appreciably lower their standards of achievement. They do not think of their age first and of their activity second, but just carry on living.

In our society few people work beyond their physical capacity. Those who do, or those whose lives are too stressful or too boring have, at any age, every right to want to ease their burden. But those who are reasonably fit, who live reasonably challenging, reasonably relaxed lives have no need to curtail their activities or interests just because they are getting chronologically older. The longer they continue living as before, the longer will they remain fit. If any activity becomes too strenuous for one reason or another their bodies will let them know soon enough. The thing to do is to check with the doctor to see whether any specific cause is responsible. There may be no reason to relinquish the activity, but simply to take a smaller dose of it, or to take it at a slightly slower pace.

Sometimes external events occur which force inactive people to do more. They usually cope and feel the benefit of being more active. It may be the arrival of a grandchild, the need to take care of a frailer person, or the chance to take up a hobby. But to wait for an external event to trigger off greater activity is too haphazard a way to foster our vitality. We should see to it ourselves that we do not stagnate.

We should consider taking up new pursuits and interests as we grow older as a refreshment and an enrichment of our lives. It would not be wise to start rock-climbing, at any age, if one is not in peak condition. But a whole range of activities can be enjoyed at whatever age we start, walking, swimming, golf, gardening, bird-watching, to name but a few.

A study was recently concluded, in which a group of elderly people had pursued an extensive programme of physical exercises. They began at an average age of 60, and their progress was followed for the next ten years. They were not athletes, but ordinary folk. They all progressively improved their performance over this period of training. At 70 they were physiologically fitter (one might say 'younger') than they were at 60.

It is therefore a misconception to regard calendar age as a limiting factor in what we are capable of doing.

PART II

(b) The mental component of life

9
Regarding Life as a Continuum

Corner-stone for a positive view of ageing
In our society we are confronted with so many subdivisions and categories of people. There are the infants, the pre-school children, the pre-teens, the teenagers, the young marrieds, the middle-aged, the over-forties, the pre-retirement group, the retired, the over-sixties, the ageing, the elderly, the aged, the old. These subdivisions may be necessary for purposes of administration and organization of various social services; they certainly seem to create special targets for commercial enterprise. But what does all this do for us as individuals? Does it help us in any way to orientate ourselves in our life? I believe that it certainly does that, but not at all positively or helpfully. It presents us, albeit subliminally, with a view of life as a series of 'stages', with milestones marking the boundaries between them. There is nothing wrong with this view of life applied to the period between birth and the physical attainment of adulthood: here progress and expansion are obvious and hope abounds. But problems soon begin: even teenagers may have anxieties of passing the dread age of twenty, beyond which they envisage entering the ranks of the 'have-beens'. And anxieties build up in this way as life goes on. We dread the Rubicons before we come to them: the age of forty, the menopause, retirement, senility and so on.

We need to be liberated from this dread of milestones, and to judge the quality of our life at any time on its own merits. Dr Benjamin Spock in his book on child care based his whole approach to the welfare of mother and child on such liberation of the parents from preconceived ideas about the 'milestones' which children were supposed to pass at some uniform, preordained ages. Dr Spock urged the parents to understand that there are fairly broad limits within which a growing child reaches various stages of development. There is so much individual variation that each child's progress should be judged on its own merits rather than on some canons of what is supposed to be 'normal' for his particular age. This attitude would be of benefit to us throughout life.

Our lives may be likened to a river, starting from small beginnings, and gathering volume as it flows through different landscapes. We develop and evolve throughout life, but we remain our essential selves.

This brings me to what I believe is a corner-stone for developing a sound, positive and healthy philosophy of ageing. The crux of the matter is to view life as a continuum. That is what many people who are chronologically old, but who are full of vitality, feel instinctively. They enjoy life as it comes. They do not hanker after recapturing their youth. Since they do not view life as a series of stages, they escape the sense of impoverishment as each milestone is passed, and avoid feeling that something of life has been jettisoned.

Life lived as a continuum is a garnering of enriching experience. It becomes a process of addition rather than of subtraction; of a growing maturity rather than of a loss of youth; of evolution rather than dissolution. It removes the pernicious, if subconscious, obsession with calendar age which precludes some of us from learning new things, or undertaking new tasks, or taking a new interest in the world around us. The less obsessed with age we are, the more readily we shall go on participating in life. We thus avoid the vicious circle of less participation, less physical and mental activity, more apathy, etc. – all of which does lead to physical and mental decline, at any age.

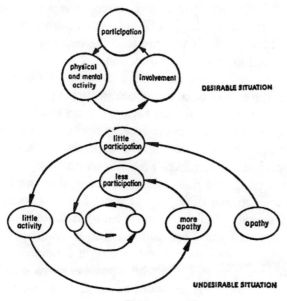

Figure 2

It is true that our society does not always encourage us to participate. Retirement arrangements are often too rigid. There is insufficient provision of alternative opportunities for paid or voluntary work after retirement or for housewives whose families have left home. This situation deprives the older citizens of a chance of fulfilment, and it deprives society of a vast reservoir of experience, skill and understanding. Some people are fortunate enough to have created for themselves a new lease of life; I can cite two cases as illustration. A retired business man has positively blossomed out now that he applies his business acumen through a voluntary organization to advising people on taxation and financial problems. A lady whose family has grown up trained, and is now active, as a marriage guidance counsellor with benefit to her clients and to herself. One hopes that the increasing numbers of people who are retired, but by no means decrepit, will organize themselves in an effective way to promote post-retirement activities. It will be pressure from within this section of society which will produce the necessary rethinking and lead to action in the right direction.

People accumulate wealth with satisfaction, enjoyment and pride. Years, too, can be accumulated in such a positive way. If we look at life as a continuum then whatever each year brings leaves a deposit of greater experience, greater confidence, greater knowledge, more interests, more appreciation and under-standing, and more tolerance. To put it another way: instead of looking at ageing as a diminishing of our quality, we can con-sider it as we consider the ageing of wine. The best qualities and the special excellence of the wine are brought about by allowing it the necessary *time* and providing it with the right conditions. To a large extent we have to create the right conditions for our-selves – and we have to begin with a positive attitude to life. In our progress – and I use the word advisedly – through life, the emphasis of our values shifts. In earlier years we measure our worth by the outward signs of success; in later years our value lies in the quality of our person, enriched by a long life.

10
Avoiding Some Pitfalls

'Opting out'

If we accept that life may be regarded as a continuum, certain practical consequences follow. Basically, the excuse disappears for 'opting out' of further development on grounds of age. We remain capable of further development, of acquiring new interests, attitudes, tastes or even prejudices. To opt out may not be our deliberate choice, but we get out of the habit of welcoming new things, because in our middle years we are too preoccupied with a limited number of activities. Some of us are busy gaining bread and getting on in our jobs; others are busy bringing up their families, keeping house or doing good works. Whatever our preoccupations they will take up a great deal of our time, thoughts and interest, and extraneous things have little chance of engaging our attention. While thus preoccupied we do not notice any particular lack; in fact there is often too much to do. When our preoccupations recede we may then feel that content has largely gone out of our life as well, and we are left impoverished.

There are some fortunate people among us who avoid such a situation by managing to be alert to the world around them. They respond to it with interest and enthusiasm even through their busy years. They then have plenty to fall back on when the main 'business' of their middle life is over. Their vitality often blossoms out precisely when many less fortunate people settle down to a humdrum inner life in a humdrum outer setting. One knows of elderly people who take up hobbies, who study, who travel, who read contemporary literature, or listen to contemporary music. They are people of today, who do not pattern their life on their calendar age. They have a wealth of life behind them and a full life ahead of them. They enjoy both vitality and maturity.

There are also many other people who live according to patterns hallowed by time and custom, and who run the risk of developing what may be termed 'mental arthritis'. This is a difficult condition to treat once it has set in; but not a very difficult one to prevent. Essentially, this condition is what we are pleased to call, rather smugly, 'getting set in our ways'. We often accept this as a natural consequence of getting older.

'Mental arthritis' follows from 'opting out' of further development beyond some standard reached in our middle years. It is a pity that whereas social stigma attaches to those young in years who 'opt out', no such stigma attaches to those who do so in middle or later life. We think it unnatural and reprehensible if youngsters drag out a listless existence, denying themselves every opportunity of developing their potential. It is equally sad and reprehensible when middle-aged or older people do not participate in the life and thought of the present with a sense of belonging to the present. After all, there are worthwhile and beautiful things around us always.

In 'opting out' we seek a refuge from the present by harking back to the past. This is a barren occupation. *Our* past is mostly a bore to everyone but ourselves, for it is an inward-looking aspect, and inward-looking people are, naturally enough, left to themselves. Such concentration on our past only happens when there is not enough *present* to fill the vacuum. The present is always there, but we need to be friendly to it and welcome it into our lives. Exciting things and good things are happening in our times. Our past may be boring but not the past of mankind.

It is our good fortune that we can enrich ourselves from either source.

The origins and the hazards of 'mental arthritis'

The origins of 'mental arthritis' go back to our youth. Its progress goes somewhat like this : when we are growing up the setting of our lives forces us to be alert to many things. We are listening, reading, learning – we are acquiring a vast number of impressions. By the time we reach 30 or so, we have had a chance to decide that we like, and enjoy, and appreciate some things more than others. We have acquired 'tastes' and 'views' and 'attitudes'. Underneath, we feel rather pleased about this, for it indicates to us that we have really grown up. We know what we like and what we do not like. But we are apt to enjoy this feeling far too long. A consolidation of some years is fine; but with time the tastes and views and attitudes tend to harden into fixed or outdated ideas and prejudices. 'Mental arthritis' has arrived on the scene.

This arrival poses a real threat to our vitality in later years. It blocks mental flexibility – a quality of mind which is the best insurance of continuing vitality. With flexible minds we can adapt to changing circumstances, whether personal, professional or social. We can then welcome a change of role, at home or at work. We can better participate in the changing world around us, and so avoid having to fall back on our past to provide content for our life.

Protection from 'mental arthritis'

Two of the ways in which we can protect ourselves from developing 'mental arthritis' are a review of personal attitudes, and achieving real contact with younger people.

It is salutary to make a conscious effort to review our mental postures, tastes and prejudices from time to time. If we loathe the music of Wagner, for instance, it is worthwhile to go and hear a Wagner opera again with a 'fresh ear', with an open mind. It may be that we have not read a contemporary novel in ten years simply because we disliked a book then in vogue. It is worthwhile to read a few new books and form some fresh (good or bad) opinions about contemporary writing. If we have always voted for one political party, it is worthwhile to read without prejudice about the policies of the rival parties. If we have read the same newspaper for many years, it is refreshing to read a different one from time to time. If we bother in these ways we are unlikely to become inflexible in our minds and rigid in our habits.

I cannot stress enough the *mutual benefit* of people of different ages living in contact with one another. I do not mean just inhabiting neighbouring houses or flats, but communicating with one another, doing things together, helping one another when necessary. The older people can very often contribute as much as the younger ones in such a symbiotic relationship.

In this connection I should like to mention a most interesting development. An experimental project in Syracuse, N.Y., was realized in which a building is used so that one half of it is occupied by college students and their young families, and the other half by retired people. The project has proved a great success and an enrichment for both kinds of tenant. The younger ones turn to the older people for advice, for help with personal problems, for help with their young children, and so on. The older ones call upon the younger ones for companionship, for information, for help with various odd jobs, etc. There is a flow of human communication and involvement. The 'generation gap' disappears when there is such viable mutual contact. The inhabitants of the building have come to know one another as *people*, regardless of their ages. As a side issue it is probably a salutary experience for the older people to realize again just how many problems young persons have to contend with. This arrangement is, in a sense, a return to the situation which still exists in Southern Europe and in most developing countries, where the older people are an integral part of the extended family and of the community.

Some years ago a television film showed a contrasting social arrangement in Sweden. Sweden provides splendid social services and adequate pensions. The film showed beautifully run old age homes, comfortable surroundings and modern amenities. But the older people living in these communities are isolated from the mainstream of life. Everything is done for *them*, but they have no opportunities to *give* anything to anyone. They lead materially comfortable, but inwardly impoverished and dispiriting lives.

It is generally a dispiriting situation when elderly people are in touch predominantly with others of their own age. There is too little opportunity then to come across fresh situations and attitudes to life. It may feel 'safer', more comfortable, or be less trouble to be surrounded by one's contemporaries if we envisage an element of competition with the young, but it is far less enriching and vitalizing. In the United States some elderly people form exclusive settlements where only the retired are welcome. Here again they live in isolation from the mainstream of life. To my mind this is 'opting out'. However youthful their pursuits, it is a retreat from challenges and a refusal of the chance to foster and develop vitality in calendar old age. Instead, it seems to me that such isolationism is a surrender to the fallacy that 'old people' are a species different from 'people'.

'You can't teach an old dog new tricks'
There is another factor which too often prevents us from trying to expand our interests and activities as we grow older. This is the widely held view that our *ability* (not our readiness or our opportunities) to change, to absorb new ideas, to learn new skills, diminishes with age. This contention is suspect, for our capacity remains potentially there into extreme old age. There are many elderly people who succeed in new ventures, which

make demands on their mental abilities. A grandmother first learned to drive at 65, and progressed so well that she qualified for an Advanced Motorist's certificate. Another lady, aged 93, passed stiff public examinations in the Russian language, which she began to learn at 90. A lady of 96 has just published a book about her childhood in Victorian England: she had the ability and the courage to venture into writing in her 90s. Such examples could be multiplied manyfold. I doubt whether many people who assert that 'you can't teach an old dog new tricks' do so after having tried really hard to learn something new. I fear that this saying is repeated more on hearsay than from first-hand experience.

So-called scientific reports and opinions claiming that mental performance declines with age are often accepted uncritically. For example, a recent article in the press discussed how in a number of professions peak performance occurs at particular ages. The ages were given with uncalled-for precision: for instance 34, rather than 30–35, and so on. On the other hand it was not mentioned how the data were obtained. A neat graph illustrated how in each profession performance rose to a peak at a particular age and then fell away. To an uncritical reader this would provide, by supposedly scientific methods, convincing and dispiriting 'proof' that we all get 'past it' as we grow older. But to a critical mind it provides no proof at all.

To begin with, one cannot rely on data if one does not know by what method they were arrived at. Also, any data taken from a number of individuals will at best represent only an approximation, unless the number of individuals examined is very *large*, and the variation within this large group is very *small*. To illustrate how misleading the conclusions of such reports can be, let us suppose that data were obtained from people in academic professions and were based on the dates when they published the results of their researches. Many factors in addition to the work done and age are here involved. At the beginning of a career people have strong motivation to work very hard, to get ahead in their jobs, and to publish their findings. At some later age they achieve their greatest productivity, and may be promoted to a more senior position. They will then be required to administer and organize and supervise other people's work. They sit on committees, and otherwise broaden their activities. All this leaves much less time and opportunities for being 'productive' in the same sense that they were some years earlier. All this relates to the professional side of their life. Their personal affairs are also relevant. People acquire families, interests, responsibilities, and these fragment their attention, time, and effort. There is no harder working or more productive specimen than a keen Ph.D. student in a high-powered University department. But he is not normally burdened with too many extraneous personal responsibilities. Professionally his time is devoted entirely to his work on his project. With all these factors playing a part the meaning of 'peak performance' becomes blurred, and the above report becomes a very unimpressive document. The only really meaningful comment in the report was the forecast that 'exceptions' will form the largest category, when the methods of collecting and analysing data become really precise and refined. In other words, in a really good investigation no firm conclusions relating to age become possible. This tallies with general observations, for it is very obvious that there is individual variation of vigour and of performance in any age group, including the very old, if we take enough factors into consideration.

Calendar age is too often paraded in isolation, and conclusions are glibly drawn that it is age itself which affects our performance or our abilities.

A possible reason why some older people take longer to learn new tasks

Various studies have shown, at different times, that older people are perfectly capable of learning new tasks, and of acquiring new skills, but that they usually take longer than younger people to do so. This observation has been taken as a sign that older people 'slow down'. Recently the ability of elderly people to memorize and recall new information was exhaustively tested at the Duke University Center for the Study of Aging and Human Development. It was found, as before, that the older subjects needed longer than the younger ones to perform their tasks. The reason for this time lag was then investigated. It turned out that the slowing down was caused by *anxiety*: the older group aimed less at achieving success than at avoiding failure. Blood tests provided biochemical evidence that the older subjects were undergoing the physiological equivalent of anxiety, but *without being consciously anxious*. Drugs which counteracted the anxiety helped them to improve their performance. The investigators suggested that what had initially slowed down the elderly subjects was not so much their age, as their *attitude* to their age. They had not *expected* to be able to perform the task set for them. Such subconscious anxiety may well be widespread, and may hamper people's performance at new tasks, even under non-test conditions. These experiments suggest that a poorer *performance* by an elderly person does not necessarily stem from a lack of *ability*.

Running out of ideas
People often say that when they were in their 20s they were full of ideas, but that this is no longer so now that they are older. Granted, they were full of ideas. But were not many of these ideas half-baked? As one set of ideas was relinquished without ever having been tested out, it was replaced by another set. To have a bagful of jigsaw puzzle pieces is not in itself valuable, if one has not checked whether they actually fit together to produce a picture. As we grow older more of our ideas have to be put to the test, and so we are forced to develop the habit of smartly dismissing the half-baked ones. This constitutes better judgment. Creative thinkers, like Bertrand Russell, were not hampered by

age. And many more ordinary people only begin to have worthwhile ideas in their 30s or 40s, when they have built up a sufficient
foundation of knowledge and experience.

Setting our sights too low

In considering what is an appropriate standard of performance
for people in their later years we tend to set our sights too low.
We look at elderly people around us who have not done anything
new or challenging for years, and we are satisfied that this is normal
'for their age'. We would not dream of looking at a group of not
very bright, unambitious, unsuccessful people in their 30s and
conclude that their situation is normal for their age. We would
still assume that younger people should strive and advance. We
make no such assumption about older people. But there are
plenty of examples of older people, who aim high and achieve
success. It is these people we should take as models for ourselves.
Their vitality is unimpaired and their alertness is sustained by
their activities. Sir Francis Chichester set himself the task of
sailing round the world at an age (65) when most people would
do nothing more adventurous than to dig a little in their garden.

Recreation

To conclude this chapter I want to say a little about the danger
of neglecting recreation. In this context I use the word both in
the sense of refreshment, and in its literal one of 're-creation'.
Essentially, any activity which is not routine for us may be
termed recreation. For sedentary people it may be chopping
wood; for a woodcutter it may be a quiet hour listening to the
radio; for solitary people it may be a trip to town; for a school-
teacher it may be a quiet walk in the fields. The essence of
recreation, in both its meanings, is *change*. In this respect, the
old saying that 'a change is as good as a rest' carries a good deal
of wisdom. To remain vital and flexible our minds and our
bodies need refreshment, they need change, new activities, new

impressions. When we reach maturity it is up to us to watch out lest we lose flexibility. For the impetus will not come from the outside. We are excused 'getting set in our ways'. But if we harden into inflexibility, we are heading towards decline into 'old age' – a sad process, but one which should not be blamed on the passage of time.

PART III

Some Practical Suggestions for the
Older Person on How to Maintain and
Improve Physical and Mental Vigour

11
Ageing Well

The earlier parts of this book served to provide the foundations of a reasoned, and rational, approach to the problem of ageing well. We have seen that improvement in health and vitality are real possibilities, and Part III deals with some relevant practical suggestions.

What we make of our 'old age' is largely up to us: it can be wretched, it can be verdant. But verdant old age doesn't happen of itself; we need to work at it. Practically speaking, what we need to do is to develop a positive attitude to living. We need to look after our health sensibly, without becoming hypochondriacs. The question of positive health embraces proper nutrition, sufficient exercise and mental stimulation. Emotionally we can be enriched and enlivened through good relationships with other people. These topics are discussed in this part of the book. I do not propose to give a digest of geriatric conditions; of calorie-values of foodstuffs; of the relative merits of Yoga, aerobics, and other exercises; or of the pros and cons of adult education and psychotherapy.

To have to work at the quality of our life may sound a daunting prospect. But, then, we all have to do it all the time. Children and young people have to study to achieve a better 'chance in life'; in middle years people strive hard to further their ambitions and achievements. In later life too many of us are content to strive for nothing. But we shall achieve a better life simply through modifying some habits which may have hardened over the years, and which become progressively more detrimental to us. It is from this point of view that the above aspects of positive health are dealt with. The problem of having sufficient exercise, for instance, arises from a diminution from childhood onwards of what is termed 'kinesophilia'. Kinesophilia is a term used for the instinctive need for movement, which is expressed in the restless mobility of children. They cannot keep still, and their physiological need for exercise is thus amply fulfilled. Why kinesophilia diminishes as we reach adulthood is not known; it would form a fascinating subject for research. The cultural patterns of present-day life help to diminish it further. Hence the situation is such, that adults, young and old, have to take conscious steps to make sure that they have sufficient physical activity.

For physical activity, therefore, we have, at least in childhood, an internal force which provides the necessary impetus. It is largely external forces, however, which operate in childhood, youth, and in middle years to furnish us with mental stimuli. In later years such external forces as educational pursuits, professional occupation, etc., recede. So the need then arises, if we want to keep our minds alert and our imagination lively, to work at finding fresh stimuli. The first hobby or pursuit that we take up may not succeed in this respect, and we need to 'shop around' for new interests. The very process of 'shopping around' for new skills and for new knowledge is in itself a refreshment.

We need to shape our daily life so that *each day* we do something positive to exercise our bodies and involve our minds. We should get about. We should read, listen, talk.

The purpose of all this beavering away at the quality of our life is not to recapture youth, or to become overblown boys and girls. Few of us, I dare say, would want to recapture the doubts, lack of self-confidence, lack of perspective, lack of experience, of youth. The aim is to enjoy our maturity, to extend our vitality, and thus to age well.

12
Some Guidelines on Positive Health

This chapter is not intended to serve as an exhaustive catalogue, or a blueprint, of measures for achieving positive health. It is intended to provide some simple guidelines, based on present-day thinking. The basic premise is very simple: it is sensible to look after your health as you grow older, without becoming morbidly preoccupied with it.

The value of medical check-ups
It is quite natural that you may have some anxieties about your health as you grow older. It is therefore very important to establish a good, open relationship with your doctor. Tell him that you wish to keep as well, fit, and independent as possible, for as long as possible. Ask him to give you a periodic check-up and to advise you on the best way to achieve this aim. You will not be trespassing on your doctor's time with such a request. On the contrary, the value of a periodic check-up is that it may uncover some minor condition, or disability, which can be easily put right at that stage. Minor ailments and disabilities, if neglected, may multiply or develop into more serious illnesses. It then becomes harder to treat them. For example, if you have had a cough for a few weeks, it is better to trouble your doctor about it, than to leave it for months or even years and then perhaps end

up with chronic bronchitis. If you have a bit of a backache, or some stiffness in any joint, it is better to see the doctor, to have some X-rays taken and to have the right treatment prescribed at an early stage. Otherwise you might simply move about less and less because of the discomfort and decline into increasing immobility with its attendant threats to health and independence.

Visits to the doctor

If you do not feel well and decide to go and see your doctor, there are one or two things which you can do to make it easier for him to help you properly.

The doctor needs to have as much relevant information as possible from you, before he can form a clear picture of your complaint. I do not mean that you have to tell him a long or elaborate story when you come to see him. But you need to tell him *enough* relevant facts. He may not have the time to put a great many questions to you to winkle these facts out and so to know how best to help you. For instance, supposing a very close friend of yours has died. You are sad and depressed, and cannot sleep properly. If you come and tell the doctor: 'I have been sleeping badly,' he may be too busy to probe into the reasons for your insomnia. He will simply write out a prescription for sleeping tablets, which will help you sleep, but you will still feel depressed, dejected and listless. If, however, you tell the doctor: 'I have recently lost a very close friend, and I have been sleeping badly,' he will instantly know that you are suffering from (medical) depression. He will be able to treat the cause, and not merely the symptom, and will prescribe an anti-depressant drug.

Quite often people are worried about some particular disease: they may have a phobia of cancer, or heart disease, or mental illness. They may not voice this fear at all to their doctor, but will go to him under the pretext of some symptoms. These may be psychosomatic, i.e. they are an expression of anxiety and not the result of attack by a germ of a virus or the effect of a physical disorder. What is the doctor to do in such a case? He will do his best to treat the symptoms, which may clear up. Others may appear in their stead, because fear – the underlying cause of the anxiety – has not been removed. Here again it would be so much better for the patient to tell the doctor quite openly about the fear, and to ask him for proper information and reassurance. To have the symptoms checked in the light of this knowledge would be much more meaningful for the patient and for the doctor.

Health surveillance clinics

The preventative aspect of positive health may be dealt with very effectively by special clinics for older people. They are unfortunately still woefully few, but it is my fervent hope that their number will increase.

These clinics offer an approach basically similar to that of the baby clinics which have become an integral part of child health and welfare services, and which greatly helped to produce much healthier generations of children. Baby and child clinics are very different establishments from hospitals for sick children. The clinics keep an eye on normally *healthy* children. Their progress is noted, and, in case of any deviation from health, a competent staff can advise the parents to take their child to a specialist or to a hospital. Exactly the same principle operates in a clinic for the elderly, such as the one in East Kilbride in Scotland. Here reasonably fit, elderly people come for an initial thorough medical examination, and thereafter return for regular check-ups. Advice is given on general topics, such as nutrition, and exercise. Any domestic, social or financial problems are discussed. If necessary arrangements are made to consult a social welfare worker. If any disease is found in the course of examination, the elderly person is referred to a specialist or for appropriate treatment in hospital. Dental problems and those of hearing and eye-sight are sorted out.

These clinics do not usurp the place of the general practitioner, but they act as a health surveillance centre. If there were a network of such clinics throughout the country much pressure would be taken off individual doctors and hospital outpatient departments. The clinic could detect minor ill health, minor disabilities or early signs of disease. These are often neglected by the elderly, who mistakenly accept them as inevitable accompaniments of ageing, and can deteriorate into chronic conditions which the doctors are then asked to treat. Regular attendance at a clinic would provide an element of continuity in health care, and serve to give support and reassurance to the elderly person.

Criteria of health

There is another point about health. At any age, you are either in Good Health, or Middling Health, or Ill Health. 'You are in good shape considering your age,' is an ambiguous statement. It presumes that there are some specific standards of good health at *particular* ages. But the notion of age is, strictly speaking, irrelevant to considerations of health. For nobody would regard anaemia as 'bad health' in a child of 7, but 'good health' in a child of 10. Similarly, we are less prone these days to regard raised blood pressure as 'bad health' in a man of 30 but 'normal' in a man of 70. There is only bad health, or good health. Bad health should be prevented, and its causes treated, whatever the age of the patient. This of course is precisely what geriatricians are doing. They treat, cure and rehabilitate chronologically elderly patients. They succeed, as do paediatricians or obstetricians in their particular specialities, against the odds of deterioration, infection or physical damage, if these are not overwhelming. It just does not happen that in a group of elderly people suffering from a particular condition of a similar severity, all those *below* a certain age will respond well to treatment, whilst all those *above* that particular age will fail to respond. Those who will respond best to treatment will not necessarily be the youngest ones, but those who have the best constitution or who are the fittest.

Depression

It is most important not to neglect the fact that after every illness we go through a period of depressed vitality. Post-influenza depression is as real an affliction as influenza itself. It may make us stay listlessly at home for several weeks: we do not get out of doors as we should, filling our lungs with fresh air and our blood with oxygen. Depression can be slight, it can be severe; it is always undesirable. It can, however, be very successfully treated by a variety of drugs.

To illustrate a very striking example of depression, complicated by several other conditions. A lady in her 70s had rheumatoid arthritis, and was in great pain, very stiff and unable to look after herself. For several years she had various treatments in and out of hospital. Eventually the rheumatoid arthritis improved a great deal. She then most unfortunately contracted shingles and was again ill and in pain. She could not hold any food down, lost a great deal of weight, and eventually became mentally confused. It seemed that she was now in a state of senile dementia, an irreversible condition. She had been most thoroughly investigated at various times and no malignancy or any other lesion was ever found. It was her good fortune that investigations were continued. It was discovered that she was severely anaemic, and her blood responded well to the appropriate treatment. But she was still confused and 'not herself'. She was then given anti-depressant drugs and these produced the most splendid results. She improved in every way, began to eat properly and put on weight. The most striking feature of all was the return, as it were, of her 'self'. She is now fully oriented in space and time, takes an interest in life, is in touch with her friends, writes letters, goes shopping and so on. She *is* her own former self and is now out of hospital.

If severe depression can cause such profound mental and physical deterioration, then lesser degrees of depression can 'dampen' vitality and well-being. This can happen as we grow older not specifically because of our age, but because of various factors: retirement, boredom, isolation, financial worries, illnesses, fears, bereavements. If you have had an illness, a bereavement, are lonely, feel afraid, have had an accident or an upset – do see your doctor, tell him about it, and let him see whether you are, in fact, suffering from depression. In this context depression is not just a mood, but a debilitating medical condition which does respond to treatment. Do not ignore it: when you are depressed you tend to neglect everything, and it needs an effort of will even to go and see a doctor. But it is most necessary to do so.

The need for attention to eye-sight and hearing

The more contact you have with the world, the healthier it is for you. You are more involved with life. There is more mental input, leading to more response and to more vitality. This stimulus may in fact occur in a circumscribed environment. A recluse can be involved in a whole world, without speaking to a soul, if he happens to be passionately interested in some topic and spends his days reading and thinking about it.

To keep in contact with the world you need the use of your senses. You need to see, to hear, to feel by touch. It may seem obvious that you have to ensure that your eyes and ears function properly. And yet many of us resist this idea and thus do not benefit from modern aids.

Eye-sight

Spectacles are so much a part of life these days, that most people do not hesitate to have their eyes checked periodically, to order the right glasses and to wear them at appropriate times. The use of spectacles puts the onus for better vision fairly and squarely on the possessor of the eyes behind the spectacles. It has nothing to do with your family, friends, or casual contacts. This situation contrasts with that of hearing, as we shall see later.

There are two conditions about which people sometimes worry: cataract, which is an opacity of the lens of the eye, and glaucoma, a disease which leads to an increase in the pressure of the fluid in the eye. Neither condition results in loss of vision if it is not neglected. It is a good idea to have your eyes checked regularly for these conditions. Either your doctor or an eye specialist will be able to do this for you. Any deterioration of vision or pain in the eyes should of course be reported to your doctor as early as possible.

Hearing

Loss of hearing is usually a gradual process, and its progress is not associated with as much helplessness as is loss of vision. So the incentive to seek help with our hearing is less than with failing eye-sight. Another point about hearing is that it involves other people since it is a mechanism of communication. People whose hearing is faulty sometimes fail to seek timely help, because they ascribe their inability to hear properly to the poor enunciation of those around them.

The disability of less than perfect hearing is a peculiarly unfortunate one, in that it often produces a reaction of irritation or impatience in those with whom the person comes in contact, instead of eliciting sympathy and concern, as lack of good vision does. This reaction compounds the misery and often contributes to the afflicted person's tendency to withdraw from human contact. Such withdrawal isolates and it erodes the habits of listening and of contributing to a conversation.

Modern hearing aids do not restore perfect hearing but they ameliorate the situation. Their success depends on the cause and the degree of the loss of hearing. In any event it is of the greatest importance that if your hearing seems to be less acute than formerly you should consult a doctor. If a hearing aid is thought to be appropriate, then acquire one and *use* it. This point, though obvious, needs some emphasis. Hearing aids are not something you can just put on and forget about, like a hat. You will need to adjust to the increased volume of sound around you, which you have perhaps not been aware of for some time. The correct volume at which the hearing aid is set must be worked out by you for individual situations. Even the feel of a plastic mould in the ear is a factor which you have to get used to. Most hearing aid consultants are perfectly happy for their clients to come back again and again to have their ear-moulds modified, to make the fit as comfortable as possible. But it is absolutely of no use to acquire a hearing aid, to put it on once or twice, and then not to bother wearing it. Aesthetically, modern aids are far less conspicuous than any spectacles. They are likely to become as socially acceptable as glasses or as dentures. The extraneous noise which you become aware of when using a hearing aid is often a nuisance. But people with normal hearing have to pay a similar penalty for the privilege of hearing what is of interest or importance to them.

I know it is easy to give advice, and far more difficult to accept or follow it. It is sad but true that people will not consistently remember to speak clearly and loudly. So it is largely up to you to make the effort of using the aid. You can say quite openly that you do not hear well and ask the indulgence of those around you for this. Above all do not withdraw from human society. It may be less trouble to you to avoid people, but it will impoverish your life. After all most people are sympathetic when they realize that a person is handicapped in some way, even if they do not always remember to act more considerately.

Care of the feet
If we have good feet we shall not think twice about going out to meet friends, or going shopping, or taking a walk. Good feet are

of the essence for sufficient mobility. If our feet hurt our will to move is sapped. Unfortunately many people suffer from such conditions as fallen arches, callouses, bunions, corns, ingrowing toe-nails, or the effects of wearing uncomfortable shoes. Most of these conditions can be alleviated. The services of a chiropodist are available, and should be made use of as soon as discomfort is felt. If the joint of the big toe is badly deformed it is well worthwhile to consult your doctor. There are orthopaedic procedures which successfully correct this painful condition. It is, of course, wise to buy well-fitting shoes. Slippers do not support the feet properly, and this distorts the action of the joints, tendons and ligaments, which help to bear the weight of the body. So do not walk about in bedroom slippers during the day, even when you are not going out and are not expecting visitors. Wearing slippers is also bad for morale; it makes you feel sloppy.

13
Nutrition

General remarks

This chapter is not intended as a guide to the constituents of various foodstuffs, or as a discussion of the myriad diets which are in vogue. It deals with some general principles of nutrition and of dietary habits in the context of their usefulness for positive health.

Proper nutrition should supply us with all the substances necessary for maintaining our health and strength and for providing energy, without making us overweight. What type of foods we eat and how much we eat are both important, if we want to safeguard ourselves against four main hazards of incorrect nutrition, *viz*. obesity, malnutrition, undernutrition, and an increased risk of developing atherosclerosis.

Obesity

It is possible that your diet may become unhealthy in so far as you simply overeat. This may be because, as you grow older, you restrict your physical activities. Less physical activity means that less food is needed by the body. Any excess of food you eat is not then used by the body, but is deposited as fatty tissue, and obesity results. There may be other reasons for overeating, such as boredom or worry; the result will be the same. In any event the cause of obesity is always the same: too much food.

Even mild obesity is not healthy. Extra weight puts an extra strain on the heart, on the joints, the spine and the legs. It reduces mobility because it takes a greater effort to move a greater weight. Putting on weight sets up a vicious circle: more weight, less mobility, too much food, increased weight, and so on. Obese people are also more prone to certain illnesses, e.g. atherosclerosis, varicose veins, diabetes. They take longer to recover from surgical procedures. They have to pay higher life insurance premiums.

Therefore, to watch your weight is a positive health measure. Get your weight down to its correct level. Bear in mind that weights given in charts refer to averages, and since most people are too heavy, so are these averages. To lose weight it is best to cut down on the *amount* of food you eat; especially restrict your intake of sweet and starchy foods. If you have a special passion for certain energy-rich foods, such as cheese, nuts, cream or beer, restrict these severely. When your weight has reached the correct level, keep it there by adjusting your eating-habits.

Malnutrition

It is possible to become obese and to be malnourished at the same time. A fat man is not necessarily 'well-nourished'. This apparent paradox simply means that if you eat a predominantly starchy diet, for example, you may put on a great deal of weight, but your health may suffer from a lack of sufficient protein, roughage, vitamins or minerals. If you consume mainly large helpings of starchy foods, sweet foods and sugared drinks, this may happen. Although you have plenty to eat (sufficient quantity), your health will suffer from the lack of a *balanced* diet (not the right *kinds* of food). You will feel vaguely unwell and lethargic, and your resistance to infection may be lowered. The remedy is to eat more protein, to include fresh fruit and vegetables, and to eat less starch and sugar. There is on the market a variety of properly balanced food supplement powders which contain part-digested protein, vitamins and minerals. They are easily digested, inexpensive, and valuable as an additive to your daily diet.

Undernutrition

Some older people become undernourished, because their intake of food is insufficient for their body's needs. They do not eat enough either for economic reasons or through a lack of interest. It may be that they cannot be bothered to cook for themselves alone, after perhaps a lifetime of feeding a family; or a man, left a widower, may not know how to cook. Undernutrition occurs in a surprisingly large number of cases, as some recent surveys in England and Scotland have shown. Too many people were found who subsisted on a 'diet' of bread-and-margarine and tea.

Undernutrition inevitably results in malnutrition. The structural and functional aspects of our bodies suffer. If the intake of food is insufficient, we lack the necessary protein, vitamins and minerals for normal health, and we run the risk of muscular weakness, anaemia or of sub-clinical ill health.

With protracted undernutrition people become 'old': they become weak, listless, apathetic; they move little because they have not the energy. Most likely they will not seek medical advice on their own initiative. In these situations the family, or health visitors or positive health clinics are of inestimable value, as they can find out just what constitutes the daily diet of the older person. Suitable action can then be taken, and the results will be positive and often striking. To ensure that an under-nourished person will receive proper nutrients, food supplement powders would be valuable. Instructions should be given on what constitutes a balanced diet, and some supervision that it is taken should initially be provided.

Atherosclerosis

Atherosclerosis is a degenerative disease of the arteries, in which the elasticity of the arterial wall is impaired by deposition of fatty substances, leading to formation of plaques (atheroma). Blood circulation is thus disturbed. In severe cases the artery may be obstructed, causing thrombosis. 'Coronaries' and 'strokes' are extreme cases of atherosclerotic lesions, and are both major killers in the developed countries. Even moderate degrees of atherosclerosis may lead to malfunction of the body and to physical decline. Obese people are at higher risk than those of normal weight. The underlying causes of atherosclerosis are not fully understood, but certain dietary habits seem to be associated with its prevalence. Smoking and lack of mobility also appear to be factors favouring this disease.

Certain fatty substances, cholesterol and saturated fatty acids, are believed to be harmful in the diet, if taken in excess. Foods containing these should therefore be used sparingly. A good general principle is to eat little butter, cream, lard, fat meat, fat bacon, eggs and cheese. Vegetable oils, in particular corn (maize) oil, sunflower oil or cottonseed oil, contain so-called polyunsaturated fatty acids, which are believed to be positively beneficial. It is therefore advisable to use these oils for cooking, instead of animal or dairy fats. In place of butter it is advisable to use only those margarines which contain added polyunsaturated acids, as indicated on the packaging. Ordinary margarines are made from vegetable oils by a process which *destroys* these acids.

Refined sugar (sucrose) has been suspected of playing a part in the development of atherosclerosis. Sugar, in any case, is a very fattening substance, and if we use it in tea or coffee we are liable to consume surprisingly large quantities of it, without feeling that we are 'overeating'. It has been said that we have a 'sweet tooth' because naturally sweet foods, e.g. fruit, berries and honey, are rich sources of vitamins, and our biological instinct led us to them in the remote past. Refined sugar, and sugar products, have no such value. Since they contribute to obesity they increase the risk of atherosclerosis developing. Therefore it is advisable to cut down sugar as much as possible, to sweeten drinks with sugar substitutes, and to use more honey, a more efficient sweetener than sucrose.

It has been suggested recently that Vitamin C may have a protective effect against the development of atherosclerosis. Since this substance plays an important role in many processes of the body, our diet should contain adequate amounts of it. Various fruit and vegetables are good sources of Vitamin C, but it may be advisable to take a daily dose of it in tablet form in addition, to be certain of having a sufficiently high intake of it at all times. This is a question which you may wish to discuss with your doctor.

Dietary habits

Good eating habits are the application in practice of sound nutritional principles. The word 'habits' is operative, for eating is a daily routine activity. Sensible eating, as a habit, promotes good health. A crash diet or a fad diet may alter your weight quickly, but is not a practical or desirable long-term mainten-ance measure. You should eat properly *always*. You should not eat too much, but try to keep a steady weight. A balanced diet should include meat, poultry and fish; plenty of fresh fruit, salads and vegetables; cheese, eggs and milk, in moderation. You should not eat much butter, lard, cream, fat bacon and fat meat. Use corn oil for cooking rather than dripping or lard. Cut down on refined sugar. Eat moderate amounts of bread (preferably made from the whole grain) and cereals. There are many excellent books on nutrition, diets and cooking, and it may be worthwhile to have a look at some. Basically the advice is: not too much of anything, and as much variety as possible.

Variety is important, because the taste, flavour and aroma of different foods stimulate adequate secretion of the digestive juices, which are responsible for the correct transformation and utilization of the food we eat. It is therefore not a good idea to become too routine-bound in what you eat. True, pangs of hunger will be stilled, and nourishment will be absorbed, even if you have the same food every day. But it will be altogether more enjoyable and beneficial if your palate is pleasantly surprised from time to time.

The first stage of good nutrition is proper chewing. Therefore, you need to pay due attention to your teeth or dentures, so that you are not restricted in your choice of foods. Especially ensure that you do not grow to avoid such foods as fresh fruit, salads and nuts. These foods, because of their cellulose content, provide the necessary bulk (roughage) which is essential for the proper functioning of the bowels. Adequate roughage is necessary to prevent constipation, and to ensure that the waste products of digestion do not remain too long in the large intestine, where they may ferment. The bacterial population normally present in healthy intestines depends on the right amount of roughage being provided. This so-called intestinal flora is exceedingly important because it aids the proper digestion and assimilation of nutrients, and because it synthesizes for us some of the vitamins which are essential for us.

Fluids

There seems to be a fairly widespread idea that as you grow older you should drink less fluids, presumably to spare the kidneys some of the effort involved in excretion. This is a fallacy. The kidneys can filter out the waste products and impurities from the blood much more easily if these are present in a dilute form. An efficient filtering of the blood by the kidneys is immensely important, and you help your kidneys to do this by taking in *plenty* of fluids. An amount of 3–5 pints a day is recommended.

Alcoholic drinks

It is a good idea, if you enjoy it, to take a glass of wine with a meal, or a sherry before meals, or a brandy or whisky as a night-cap. A little alcohol tends to relax you, to make a meal more enjoyable and therefore more digestible, and to embellish your daily routine in a small way. Alcohol tends to dilate the blood vessels and so to aid the circulation. Large amounts of alcohol depress the appetite, which may lead to malnutrition. Habitual heavy drinking will cause liver damage (cirrhosis), leading to impaired digestion and impaired detoxification of harmful substances in the body. The eventual outcome of this is physical and mental deterioration.

Smoking

Smoking has nothing to offer for positive health.

14
Dietary Supplements

General remarks

As we have seen, proper nutrition should supply us with the necessary proteins, fats and carbohydrates. It should also provide minerals and vitamins – the so-called accessory food factors, which play a most important role in metabolism. Evidence is accumulating that in later years the need for these substances increases. This may be due to their faulty assimilation, to defects in the ability of storing them in depots (e.g. in the liver), to changes in intestinal flora, or to other factors. A normal, balanced diet should supply an adequate amount of minerals and vitamins, but it may not meet adequately an increased need.

Vitamins are centrally placed in the biochemical scheme of things. In the organism vitamins are intimately connected with various enzyme systems. Enzymes are special proteins, which enable chemical reactions to proceed rapidly under physiological conditions; without the enzyme such reactions would occur either very slowly or not at all. Vitamins are necessary for the well-being of cells, tissues and organs, and for the metabolic balance of the whole organism.

Gross deficiencies of vitamins lead to gross, and serious, deficiency diseases (e.g. scurvy, pernicious anaemia, pellagra, beri-beri, rickets). These conditions are now very rare in the developed countries. But slight inadequacies, or imbalances, of these factors may affect adversely the functioning of the body over the years. The efficiency of metabolic processes is impaired. This is often seen in old age; it is corrected by the administration of extra vitamins. To counteract such inadequacies it is a good idea to take a daily supplement of minerals and vitamins as a prophylactic measure. Vitamin A and Vitamin D in very large doses may be harmful; others are not, and the body excretes any excess without difficulty.

Functions and sources of vitamins

Vitamin	Function	Source
Vitamin A	Physiological action concerned with normal condition of the skin and of mucous membranes, and with vision in subdued light.	Green leaves, carrots, yellow vegetables, fish liver oils, egg yolk, butter.
Vitamin B complex, consisting of:		
Vitamin B_1 (thiamine)	Part of an enzyme system concerned with the utilization of carbohydrates by living cells, and thus in the production of energy.	Widespread, but particularly in yeast, peanuts, peas, beans, lean pork, brans and germs of cereal grains.
Vitamin B_2 (riboflavin)	Has a role in the utilization of foodstuffs.	Liver, yeast, milk, eggs, green leaves, vegetables, fruit.
Niacin (nicotinic acid)	Forms part of two coenzymes, which are essential for proper carbohydrate metabolism, and other biochemical processes.	Yeast, fish, lean meat, liver, peanuts, vegetables, fruit.
Vitamin B_6 (pyridoxin)	Concerned with the utilization of proteins in the tissues.	Yeast, liver, lean meat, whole cereal grains.
Pantothenic acid	Forms part of the molecule of Coenzyme -A, which is involved in numerous biochemical processes, including the biological synthesis of fats and sterols, and the breakdown of fats.	Liver, yeast, egg yolk, milk, broccoli, molasses.

Vitamin	*Function*	*Source*
Folic acid	Important in the synthesis of nucleic acids, and in the formation of new cells in the body, in particular blood cells.	Liver, yeast, green leaves, eggs, soy beans.
Choline	Regarded as part of the B-complex, although it is synthesized in the body and is normally present in larger amounts than other vitamins. Its physiological action is concerned with the transport of fats, and with the formation of new cells in the body. A derivative, acetylcholine has an important function in nerve activity.	Egg yolk, lean meat, fish, soy beans, peanuts.
Vitamin B_{12} (cyanocobalamine)	Concerned with the biological formation of nucleic acids. Its deficiency leads to pernicious anaemia.	Lean meat, liver, fish, milk, eggs.
Vitamin C (ascorbic acid)	Functions as a coenzyme. Important in the proper functioning of the adrenal glands. It may act as a protective factor against atherosclerosis. It may raise the body's resistance to infections, including the common cold.	Citrus fruit, lettuce, tomatoes, fruit and vegetables generally.
Vitamin D	A group of related compounds, involved in the utilization of calcium and phosphorus for the formation, maintenance and repair of bone.	Synthesized in the skin under the influence of sunlight and ultraviolet rays. Liver-oils of cod and halibut.
Vitamin E (tocopherol)	Acts as an antioxidant, i.e. it helps to protect other vital substances in the body from destruction by oxidation, and combats the production of noxious substances by oxidation.	Green leaves, vegetable oils.
Vitamin K	Is the antihaemorrhagic vitamin, essential to the blood-clotting mechanism. It is also concerned in maintaining the condition of the walls of capillary blood vessels.	Green leaves; synthesized in the gut by the bacterium, *E. coli*.

Synthetic vitamins are identical in every respect with those occurring in foods. Some excellent multi-vitamin and vitamin-plus-mineral preparations are available on the market. Their contents are properly controlled, and the proportions of the various constituents are properly balanced. Using them obviates the risk of destroying some of the vitamins by cooking, or throwing them out with the vegetable water.

Minerals
Correct and balanced amounts of various minerals are essential for correct metabolism, since they enter into the composition of intra- and extra-cellular fluids, and are involved in many biochemical reactions occurring in the body. Calcium and phosphorus go to form the hard substance of bone. Iron is part of haemoglobin, the blood pigment, which occurs in the red blood cells and is responsible for the transport of oxygen in the blood. Phosphorus is an important constituent of nervous tissue. Sodium, potassium, calcium and magnesium are concerned with the electrolyte balance of the body. There are other substances, the trace elements, which are so called because they are needed in minute amounts, but without which the body cannot function properly, e.g. cobalt, copper, fluorine, iodine, manganese, molybdenum and zinc. As with vitamins it is sensible to take some mineral supplements as a prophylactic measure.

Two conditions which occur quite commonly in older people are mild forms of anaemia and osteoporosis (thinning of the bones). Anaemia may produce symptoms of listlessness, tiredness and apathy, which so many people believe to be natural accompaniments of increasing age. Very fortunately, anaemia resulting from simple iron deficiency can be readily cured by administration of iron. In former times iron therapy often had unpleasant side-effects on digestion, but modern iron-containing preparations avoid this. Anaemia is easily diagnosed by a simple blood test.

Good natural sources of iron include leafy, green and yellow vegetables; potatoes; fresh fruit, dried fruits; meat, poultry, fish, eggs; bread (enriched), whole grain cereals.

In cases of osteoporosis there is a need for extra calcium. Foods rich in calcium (e.g. milk, milk products, fruit, most vegetables and salads, and fish) can be supplemented by preparations of calcium salts.

Anabolic steroids

In later years the level of anabolic steroids, normally manufactured by the body, tends to decrease. These substances control the building-up and maintenance of muscle tissue. Their lack results in excessive breakdown (or wasting) of muscles; this accounts for much of the muscular weakness experienced by older people. Synthetic anabolic steroids are often prescribed with good effect to aid recovery from debilitating illnesses or surgical procedures, and sometimes in cases of osteoporosis. Athletes of heavy field events sometimes use, or rather misuse, these agents to increase muscular bulk and strength; this shows how potent these agents can be. For many elderly people small doses of these steroids taken intermittently, as a maintenance measure, are very beneficial. The best results are achieved in conjunction with adequate protein intake, and sufficient exercise. The protein consumed serves as a source of the raw materials (amino-acids) which the anabolic steroids help to build into the proteins of the muscles; this process is encouraged by muscular exertion. Anabolic steroids are available only on prescription.

15

Practical Suggestions on Physical Activity

General mobility

Any programme designed to improve fitness pivots on mobility. As explained in Chapter 7, it is important for us to maintain and to extend the mobility of our bodies. We recognize movement is a source, as well as the result, of vitality. We should therefore welcome it, unless our health is so poor that *any* physical exertion could endanger it further. If you have any doubts whether a gentle increase of physical activity is safe for you, do consult your doctor; he will examine you and then advise you.

We cannot hope to have the boon of sufficient physical activity if we allow our mobility to deteriorate through being too sedentary, i.e. spending too much time sitting or lying down, and driving rather than walking. If you are reasonably fit, deliberately move about as much as possible, and as frequently as possible, using as many different movements as possible. Move gently and for short periods to start with, then gently step it up. After a while you will realize that you can do more than you had thought possible, and you will feel better and will continue to feel better for it. Even if you are laid up in bed with a minor illness, do try and do some gentle exercises in bed, e.g. clench and unclench your fists, circle your feet, or draw up – then straighten – your knees. If you have a tendency to muscular or joint stiffness it is likely to worsen if you move less and less. Sufferers from these conditions know only too well that their pain and stiffness are worst when they get up in the morning – precisely after a period of bed rest, not after a period of physical activity.

It would seem a good idea to start the day with a few minutes' regular exercises. Some examples of suitable exercises are given in Chapter 16. Do these as a routine, just like brushing your teeth. Unless you are naturally at your best first thing in the morning you will find such a routine stimulating. You will extend yourself just a little, your heart and lungs and nerves will exert themselves a little, and you will be refreshed. You will be starting the day actively – and that is important, especially when there is no external reason, such as going to work, which compels you to get out of bed and out of the house. If you follow this routine with a bath or a shower, and a brisk rubbing down with a towel, you will feel invigorated. If you then take a little trouble over dressing, make-up, etc., and have a good breakfast, you will have started the day well. A shapeful morning is good for morale.

I have reservations about the widespread hankering after living in a one-storeyed house or bungalow on retirement, because 'one won't be able to manage stairs'. If you have made sure that there are no stairs, you will eventually get out of the habit of 'managing' them. This is bad health policy. Having a stairs which you are obliged to climb at least once a day, but which you can do at your own pace, is excellent exercise for the heart, the leg muscles, the knee joints and for the sense of balance. Stairs should of course be made safe to use (see Chapter 17), and if possible one should have a lavatory downstairs. You should take every opportunity to climb upstairs as a positive health measure. People of working age have long been advised to 'use the stairs instead of the lift *every time*'; to walk upstairs is sound advice after retirement as well.

The main thing to remember is that it does not matter particularly what physical activity you follow, *so long as you are active*. The more varied are your movements, the better. Avoid all jerky, too vigorous or too sudden, movements, as these may strain a muscle, pull a ligament or do some other damage. Always use gentle, springy movements. Mobility is an attribute to be treasured and cherished; its preservation deserves your attention and effort.

Walking

The general modern trend is for labour-saving, movement-saving devices. In so far as it cuts down movement in our day-to-day living this trend is deplorable. It is obviously much healthier to walk to the shops, or to the library, however slowly, than to take the car or bus. The mind boggles at people, who are not crippled, but who are not prepared to walk a few paces to their television set to change channels, choosing to install a remote-control switch. Except for getting up to the table for meals, answering the telephone occasionally and walking to the lavatory, some retired people take no exercise. They would benefit from a short walk of about half an hour before lunch. This would improve their appetite, and a snooze after lunch, if desired, would become a beneficial rest after exertion. Bad weather should not prevent anyone from having a walk every day. After all, if you return home a little cold you will soon get warm indoors; or if you get wet, you can change into dry clothes, and be none the worse for it. You can pace your walk to suit yourself. If you have got out of the habit of taking walks you may initially be rather slow, but in a month or two you should be *able* to walk faster, and longer, without difficulty.

Walking is an excellent form of exercise physiologically, and it also has several other advantages. It is a very flexible activity: you can go out alone or with someone else; you can walk slowly or quickly; you can stop whenever you like; you do not have to have any special skills or equipment, or belong to a club. Summer and winter the garden or the street or the park where you walk are always there. If you do not care for taking a walk without a specific purpose, then arrange a purpose, like shopping, buying a newspaper, going visiting or to the cinema. But walk regularly! Even if you are a little unsteady you need not feel that walking is not for you; do not be reluctant to use a stick. If your feet give you any trouble, see to them, so that you can get the maximum pleasure from walking.

Climbing

If you are not suffering from a heart condition, then there is no harm whatsoever in walking uphill, or up and down stairs. Do not be alarmed if you get a little out of breath for a few minutes after your exertion. This means that the heart and the lungs make that little bit more of an effort, and their reserve power is being increased. So do not avoid walking uphill, climbing steps or stairs, but rather take every opportunity of doing so. If you do this as slowly as is comfortable for you, and gradually do it a little faster, you will be training yourself in a very simple and effective way.

Gardening

If you have always enjoyed gardening then you are not likely to give it up just because you are getting older. It provides varied movements, some gentle some more vigorous, and has the added advantage of taking you out into the fresh air. With various modern aids it is possible to continue gardening even if you have some handicap (a bad back, or stiff joints). Rather than give up gardening because of disability it is well worth equipping your-self with such aids. Gardening is also psychologically rewarding. You are doing something constructive and creative, and you see the fruits of your efforts. If you happen to have the sort of garden which needs an enormous amount of heavy digging or other really strenuous work, then it may be worthwhile to redesign it in some way, to provide plenty of opportunity for regular exercise and yet not demand more of your strength and time than you can give to it.

Swimming

If you have for years enjoyed swimming when on holiday, do not give it up. Swimming is an excellent exercise, which benefits the muscles of the whole body, the respiratory and the circulatory systems. We weigh less when we are immersed in water; this buoyancy action enables us to achieve a positive effect with comparatively little effort. Swimming is invigorating because it is an exercise free from the discomforts of becoming too hot. A regular swimming routine would be of great benefit for keeping fit and agile. It may be a very good idea to agitate for periods of time to be set aside each week at municipal swimming pools for the use of older people. Older people may not relish using a public swimming pool when it is full of children messing about or of young adults who are boisterous. The aesthetic aspect comes into it as well; older people may be shy to parade less than perfect physiques among the slimmer, fitter youngsters.

Golf and other sports

If you have played golf, or tennis, or bowls or some other sport most of your life, then continue doing it. Even if you feel that your standard of performance is falling off, don't give it up, because the exercise is invaluable. If you have not been active in a sport, it is worth considering taking it up, when you have more spare time on your hands. Nobody is expected to be good at it right from the start, but as you progress your enjoyment will grow. Table-tennis is not an over-strenuous sport, but it certainly develops agility and coordination. The main thing is to enjoy the activity involved in a sport, rather than its competitive aspects.

Active holidays

It is a very good idea indeed to plan your holidays so that they include at least some opportunity for physical activities: walking, swimming, mountain or fell-walking, rowing, sailing or sight-seeing on foot. If you spend your holidays travelling by car or coach, and sitting on hotel terraces or on the sea-front, it will only provide a change of scenery and a refreshment in that sense. If you have in fact given up active holidays for some years, do give yourself another chance. You will very likely surprise yourself, and find that you still enjoy them. Holidays spent with younger people, one's children or grandchildren, are a great spur in this direction; even if you cannot always keep pace with the liveliest members of your group, you will still benefit from the venture.

Other activities

The activities I have dealt with above represent only a small selection of those possible. So if your personal preference is for, say, attending keep-fit classes, or ballroom dancing, these can perfectly well provide the desired physical exercise.

Training and improving performance

Whilst it is true that the performance of many older persons is at a low level, it is equally true that they can *improve* their standards of performance by simple training. This training can be achieved at any age, but the rate of improvement will vary individually, as shown by a number of recent investigations. Older people have the potential, the reserve capacity so to speak, to respond positively to increased physical activity. As shown earlier in this chapter the choice of the type of activity is up to the individual. Whatever the activity it will be gratifying if you can look back one, two or even ten years, and realize that you are now able to walk, or swim, or play tennis, or do press-ups, better than when you started, although you were then younger in calendar years. Challenging our bodies, gently and gradually, to do more, rather than less, as the years go by makes sense in this way. What is important is the physical state of our bodies, our health, not how many years that body has been alive. Activity, vitality and health are links in a chain of events, and each of these links depends on, and contributes to, the others. Activity is the only one of these factors which we can regulate *at will*, and this is the basis of self-training. You can try it out for yourself. For example, walk at your normal pace the first day and note how long it is before you begin to feel tired. Do this daily for a week and again check the time; you will most likely find that you will have walked a few minutes longer before tiring. By this little experiment you can demonstrate to yourself that your *endurance* has improved. Or try another tack: walk for the same distance each day, but each day a little faster and see how much sooner you will reach your destination point. This will show you that you can improve your *speed*. You can equally well devise other tests on this pattern. If at the end of the first week you have made little progress, carry on for a second week. Whatever the progress, it will encourage you to persevere in your training efforts. Extend this training-attitude to all your physical pursuits: if you have been gardening for four hours this week, for example, aim at five hours next week.

One can illustrate training by describing briefly a longitudinal study, to which reference was made in Chapter 8, carried out recently in Moscow, and corroborated by evidence from the U.S.A. A general regimen for a ten-year training programme was arranged for a group of ordinarily fit people, aged 51–74. It consisted of a daily routine of exercises; two one-and-a-half-hour sessions a week of group gymnastics; walking; skiing; and rambling. Periodic medical assessments included electrocardio-grams, tests of heart and lung function, and blood analyses. At the end of the study no single case of physical deterioration was observed; instead, there was generally an improvement in heart and lung function, and a striking improvement in muscular strength and coordination. One or two examples will serve to illustrate this improvement. The female subjects were all unable to do any press-ups at the beginning; on average they could achieve eight press-ups ten years later. The male subjects improved their performance by thirteen press-ups, on average, over the same period. Another exercise involved being suspended from gymnasium wall bars, raising the legs to a right-angle position and sustaining this for as long as possible. At the beginning of the programme *none* of the subjects, men or women, could perform this exercise. At the end of the training period the majority of the men, and a minority of the women, could sustain their right-angled position for longer than ten seconds. These results demonstrate clearly how real is the improvement in physical strength, agility and endurance, which can be achieved in spite of advancing years.

16
The Daily Two-dozen

General remarks

The routine of exercises, which are described here, has been selected because it provides work for a wide range of muscles, and forms a balanced set. It can be extended, if you wish to include a favourite exercise. It is composed of exercises which do not involve any violent movements, and should not produce any untoward results. This routine, regularly done, will help to keep you fit, supple and agile. Before starting on any exercise routine, it is advisable to check with your doctor. For a reasonably fit person the exercises given here should be entirely beneficial.

No exercise is of much benefit unless it is done regularly. Set aside a specific time during the day for it, such as before breakfast. If you can have a window open whilst doing the exercises, so much the better.

Start gently. All movements should be executed smoothly, slowly and rhythmically; all abrupt or jerky movements should be avoided. Step up your efforts gradually, aiming at the number of repetitions recommended. Do not be alarmed if at the end of the exercise period you are a little out of breath, say for a minute or two. If the activity causes prolonged breathlessness, or chest, joint or muscular pain, consult your doctor. If you have to interrupt your daily routine for any reason at all, try to return to your daily programme as soon as possible, again starting gently, and gradually returning to the level of exercise you had reached before the interruption.

Here is an exercise routine:

Exercises to be done while lying on your back (supine)
These should be done on your bed, or better still on the floor. Practise getting down on the floor and getting up from the floor, if you are not used to it.

1. Stretch your limbs, like a cat does on waking up.
2. Bend your toes, then straighten them out. Repeat 10 times.
3. Circle your feet at the ankles: first clockwise, then anticlockwise. In each direction 5 times.
4. Stretch your knees by pressing them towards the floor, then relax. Repeat 10 times.
5. Pull in and tighten up your buttock muscles, then relax them. Repeat 10 times.
6. Draw up your knees and together swing them first over to the right, then over to the left, as far as you can. Repeat 10 times.
7. Lift the right leg, keeping it straight, and circle it from the hip. Then repeat with the left leg. Each 5 times.
8. Draw up your knees, stretch your legs and 'bicycle' in the air. Repeat 5 times.
9. Draw up your knees, raise up your legs to a right angle, and lower your stretched legs *very* slowly to the floor. (This exercise strengthens the abdominal muscles.) Repeat as many times as you can manage, increasing gradually up to 10.
10. Keeping your arms at your sides, roll over to your right side, then over to your left side. Repeat 5 times.
11. Keeping your hands on your abdomen, and your legs stretched, raise your shoulders from the horizontal as far as you can, and repeat as many times as you can, increasing gradually to 10.

12. Raise yourself to a sitting position without raising your feet. Begin with the help of your hands; gradually progress to sitting up with your hands on your abdomen; and eventually with your hands behind your head. This is a training exercise, and at each stage you should do it as many times as you can manage, gradually increasing to 10.

Exercise to be done lying on your front (prone)
13. Place your hands under the chin. With your elbows out, and keeping them in contact with the floor, *very slowly* raise your shoulders, neck and head as far as you can *comfortably* do so, then *very slowly* lower the shoulders to your starting position, and relax. (This is a Yoga exercise and should be done very slowly, without any feeling of strain.) Gradually increase the number of times and the distance the shoulders are raised. Repeat 5 times.

Exercise to be done sitting on the floor
14. With legs outstretched in front of you slide your feet along the floor by drawing up your knees as high as you can; at the *same time* clench your fists and raise your arms straight above your head. Repeat as many times as you can manage comfortably, and gradually increase to 10.

Exercises to be be done standing
15. Stand with your back against a wall or door. Draw in your abdomen, and try to touch the vertical surface behind you with your calves, shoulder blades and back of head. Breathing normally, keep your abdomen drawn in for 1 minute. (This is an effective exercise which tones up the leg, abdomen and midriff muscles.)
16. For exercises 16–22 the starting position is with your feet apart, and holding your back and neck straight. Draw up one knee, clasping it as close to your body as you can and as

strongly as you can, with both hands. Repeat with the other knee. (Be careful, especially at first, not to lose your balance. This exercise strengthens the arm, leg and abdomen muscles, and improves the balance.)

17. Move the right hand up, from below the right knee, along the side of the body into the armpit, whilst letting the left hand descend to below the left knee. Then raise the left hand, and lower the right hand in the same way. Repeat 10 times.

18. Stretch out your arms sideways, palms facing down. Rotate the hands as far as you can manage, to have the palms facing up. (This strengthens the muscles of the forearms and of the upper arms, which tend to become flabby with most people.) Repeat 10 times.

19. Clench your fists and rest them on the front of your shoulders. Stretch your arms forward, stretching out your fingers at the same time. Return fists to shoulders. Stretch your arms and fingers sideways. Return fists to shoulders. Stretch your arms and fingers upwards. Return fists to shoulders. Bend forward from waist, letting your arms swing completely relaxed from your shoulders, like a 'rag doll'. Return fists to shoulders. Repeat the whole sequence 10 times.

20. With your hands on your hips, raise yourself on tiptoe; keep this position for a few seconds, then return your heels to the floor. Repeat 10 times.

21. Brace your shoulders back, as far as you can manage comfortably, then slump forward. Repeat 5 times.

22. Keeping your hands on your hips, take several deep breaths, letting your rib-cage expand to its fullest on each inspiration, and exhaling as much air as you can on each expiration. Let a few seconds elapse before repeating. Do this exercise slowly. Repeat 5 times.

23. Hold on to a stout piece of furniture. Keep your back straight, and raise your feet on tiptoes. Bend your knees. Try to lower your body as far as you can; you should be able

eventually to rest your buttocks on your heels. Straighten up. (You should start this training exercise gently and gradually; coax yourself to go a little lower, and to repeat it a few more times. It strengthens the leg muscles and loosens the knee and ankle joints, as well as improving agility and balance.) Repeat 10 times.

24. *EITHER* do some running on the spot, progressing gradually from a few to as many as you can do comfortably, *OR* go up and down a flight of stairs, first as slowly and as few times as you can manage comfortably (without more than a very slight breathlessness); gradually increase the speed and the number of times you can climb up and down the stairs. (This is a training exercise, which strengthens the heart.)

The whole routine takes about 15–20 minutes.

17
Safety Measures

General remarks
The number of accidents in the home, which yearly kill or maim people, is of epidemic proportions. Even more accidents occur which produce minor discomforts or disabilities. It is perfectly obvious, therefore, that due care should be taken to provide safety measures in the home, to prevent accidents. I shall list some of the more obvious measures, and doubtless there must be many more which can be taken, according to where and how you live. But the main tenet of this Chapter is that it is important to be *safety-minded*. This applies even if you live in a house you are very familiar with. It is worthwhile to go over the various rooms, kitchen, bathroom, passages, stairs, garden, etc., and to look hard where there might be a potential hazard, and then to take measures to remove it.

Steps and stairs
Stairs should have a rail along the wall, so that you can grab hold of it or of the banister, if you are not too steady on your feet, or to provide extra support. If there are awkward groups of a few steps it may be well worthwhile to substitute a ramp for them. Groups of steps leading up to the front door, or inside the house, should have a white line painted on their edges, so that it can be seen precisely how many steps there are, and where they come to an end. Stairs should be clearly lit. Two-way light switches

should be provided at the top and at the botton of each flight of stairs. Care should be taken to repair or replace worn carpeting on stairs on which you could trip up.

Floors
Floors should not be polished with slippery-finish polishes. Care should be taken not to leave any spilled water on the floor. Spilt talcum powder is a danger on the bathroom floor. Both can be extremely slippery, and can lead to bad falls. Falls in a bathroom are a special risk, if one hits the edge of the bath in the fall. Stockinged feet are slippery on all except carpeted floors.

Mats and rugs
Mats, rugs and runners should be fitted with non-slip backing. Care must be taken that the edges are not rucked up or frayed in a way which could cause you to trip over them.

Climbing on to furniture
If you have to reach up to the top of a cupboard, or hang curtains, or do anything requiring a climb on to a chair or table, make absolutely sure it is stable and is sufficiently sturdy to support your weight. The surface should be large enough to allow you some lee-way, in case you need to shift your position. Do not reach too far out to avoid the danger of the support tipping over. It is especially dangerous to climb on to polished furniture in stockinged feet. The safest thing to do is to invest in some special steps.

Generally avoid keeping your head thrown back too long, when reaching up, or looking up. Temporary 'kinking' of the arteries at the back of the neck may occur, with the risk of dizziness and a fall.

Bath or shower
Grab-rails should be provided in a suitable place on the wall alongside the bath or shower. They there serve the dual purpose

of helping a person to heave themselves up, and of providing protection against slipping on the bottom of the bath or the shower trough. There are several varieties of such rails available on the market. A suction-type rubber mat on the bottom of the bath or of the shower trough is an extremely simple, cheap and effective safety measure, and should always be used. Bath seats are useful. The temperature of the bath or of the shower should always be tested. It is safer to use a soap-on-the-rope in a shower.

Fire-guards
If you have to have an open fire, a fire-guard should be placed in front of it. Appalling burning accidents can occur in the event of a sudden unsteadiness or giddiness. Clocks or other objects should not be kept on the mantelpiece where you may get too close to the fire if you need to peer at them.

Gas leaks
If you have gas appliances in the house it is wise to have them checked for leaks, to prevent the risk of explosions.

Electrical appliances
See that all electric leads and plugs are in sound condition and have faulty ones replaced. See that electric leads do not trail across the floor, where you may trip over them. It is false economy to have weak light-bulbs; dim lights can cause accidents. It is advisable to have a light switch near the bed to avoid groping around in the dark. Take care not to touch anything electrical with wet hands.

If you have an electric blanket follow the manufacturer's advice closely on how to put, and to keep, the blanket on the bed.

Medicines

Many modern medicines are potent drugs; they are very specific and the dosage is strictly defined. It is most important, therefore, to avoid any accidental muddling up of one medicine with another. To prevent accidents see that all your medicines are clearly labelled with the *name of the drug* and *its purpose*, e.g. '*Piriton* – hayfever', or '*Mogadon* – sleeping tablet'. If necessary ask the doctor to tell you the correct names of the drugs you are prescribed; most doctors would not object to such a request if you explain. So many tablets look alike that it is easy to make a mistake, especially if you are not feeling very well, are anxious, distracted or simply sleepy. Also, if you should happen to have a different doctor attending you, or need to go into hospital, it is more helpful all round if you can tell them that you are taking, for example, drug X, two tablets a day, instead of saying vaguely you take two large white tablets a day, the little yellow one if you feel especially poorly, and the little pink one at night. Check through your medicines every so often to see that everything is properly labelled, and if there is anything which is not, throw it away. If you have medicines left over from previous illnesses, throw them away.

Getting about in wet weather

If you are using an umbrella, be careful not to obstruct your vision with it. Umbrellas made with transparent plastic are a good idea. To avoid slipping on wet surfaces (wet leaves in the autumn, slush, etc.) see that you wear shoes or boots with non-slip soles.

A traffic hazard

If you are hard of hearing, take care to cross roads where you can *see* the traffic coming from both directions.

Arrangements for obtaining help in case of illness or accident
If you live alone then it is most important that you organize some means of signalling for help if need be. This may be vital if anything serious should happen, and it will also give you peace of mind generally. There are various flashing light or buzzer devices available, with which to attract attention. Cards saying 'HELP!' can be displayed in a window. In some areas the postman is instructed to look out for such signals, and to summon help. A telephone in the house is invaluable for any emergency.

18
Mental and Emotional Aspects

General remarks

Aspects of our physical life are relatively uniform: we all digest food by the same processes; the same mechanical principles govern our movement; our metabolism proceeds by the same biochemical reactions, and so on. It is therefore feasible to give specific indications of how we can improve our health and fitness by attending to specific physical factors. This is not the case with mental and with emotional aspects of our lives. Here we come up against the real richness of human existence. There are as many mental and emotional worlds as there are people, for here individuality comes to the fore. In the picture of our inner life general principles can be regarded only as the canvas, over-laid with many layers of paint, arranged in different designs and colours. It is manifestly impossible to deal with such variety within the scope of this book. If mental and emotional factors were autonomous and divorced from the physical ones, there would be little point in attempting to deal with the general principles underlying them. But as we have seen before, the physical, mental and emotional constituents of life are inextricably linked together, and are interdependent. Therefore, mental and emotional factors have to be considered in the context of how the *total* quality of our life can be enhanced. These factors can only be considered in a very circumscribed way with the help of a few examples. We can examine what is, on the whole, of benefit to us, or otherwise. It is hoped that such general reflections will shed some light on particular situations.

Mental stimulation

Any impoverishment of our mental life is a threat of stagnation. We should therefore take every opportunity – and create opportunities – to preserve and to extend our mental involvement. The kinds of things which interest people are legion; the important thing is to keep these interests alive and to seek out others. The more active our participation in these activities, the better, for we may then derive concomitant advantages. For example, if you are fond of music you may enjoy it either through listening to records or by going to a concert. If you choose the concert not only will you have the extra delight of hearing the music 'live', but you will have had an opportunity to dress up a little, to have a journey, and to be among people drawn together by a common interest. This applies to other activities: watching football on television is not half as exciting and stimulating as being at the game itself.

Mental stimulation bears the same relationship to mental recreation and relaxation, as physical activity does to physical recreation and rest. Relaxation after mental effort or concentration refreshes us; but habitual relaxation provides little soil for ideas to grow.

It is interesting and encouraging to observe how lively and fit are many septuagenarians today, who were forced by circumstances to change their mode of life completely in their 40s. Because of the war, they had to adapt to entirely new conditions, new occupations, new attitudes. Some had to learn to live and work using a new language. Such upheaval seems to have served them as a new start in life. They had to do at 40 what most people do at 20, and they succeeded in rising to this challenge.

They certainly show no signs of 'mental arthritis'. They do not give their age much thought, but live in the present. They are years younger than their calendar age.

Advantages of contact with other age groups
Apart from the greater variety and stimulation which comes from being in touch with people of different ages, there is a particular aspect of such contacts which can be of real value to an older person. It concerns the tendency of some older people to think that nobody else has the problems which they have themselves. It is helpful for these people to realize sometimes that those who are younger are not automatically also healthier, wealthier and more carefree than themselves. Health worries exist at all ages, and in younger people may be complicated by anxiety about their family responsibilities. Financial worries dog men in their prime when they have to set up house, rear and educate children, even 'keep up with the Joneses' for career or social reasons. Loneliness is not the prerogative of the elderly: many a suburban housewife has virtually nobody to talk to all day. Husbands are not always sparkling conversationalists after a long and arduous day at work. Wives, too, are at times less than inspiring companions. There may be worries about marriage problems, about childlessness or about too many children. Younger people, as well as older ones, may suffer from disappointments, jealousies and social inadequacies. And the younger the persons, the less seasoned they are. They worry, and have not the resources and the wisdom of experience which an older person would have, to realize that most problems eventually resolve, and that one can cope with challenges and rise to meet seemingly frightening situations.

The view is often expressed that it is difficult to form new relationships when we get older. If we keep – or cultivate – human sympathy, and an open mind, why should it be difficult? Age as such is an irrelevant factor. Human sympathy is, basically, a concern for the *other* person, and this in no way depends on age. An open mind enables us to develop an interest in other people, and to store up treasure. A mind set in its ways is not necessarily a treasure house. There may be some priceless things in it, but there may also be a good deal of lesser value, which could with profit be cleared out from time to time, to admit some fresh light and air. Who knows how many priceless new things may drift into it on this current of fresh air?

It is often said that older people thrive on being needed and on being wanted. People of every age thrive on this. To be needed we have to be helpful. To be wanted we have to be pleasant.

A pleasing appearance has a part to play in how people react to us; it is, of course, also good for our morale. Our appearance is what we present to the outside world: people cannot read our thoughts or divine our feelings, but a neat and pleasing appearance signals that all is well, at least on the surface. This encourages people to approach us, and to take an interest. It may not be a laudable reaction, but people are put off by a dishevelled, unkempt or dowdy appearance. This response is true also for members of our families, and we should take especial care to please them.

Family relationships
Lack of communication between people is a characteristic of our times. Family relationships often wither because of faulty communication. In my view this happens when people abdicate from making the effort to communicate. At times older people complain, and with good reason, that their relatives or children do not understand them, or neglect them, or treat them like babies. This is a situation where much can be altered for the better if they voice clearly and calmly just what they hope for and expect from any particular relationship. This would be a positive approach, and one much more likely to produce desired results

than a silent dissatisfaction, hardening into resentment. Older people have every right to explain how they see themselves in a relationship. They are not obliged to play a part assigned to them by others, if it does not suit them. For example, they may live with a daughter, who wishes to spare them every trouble and effort, and who does not let them do anything for themselves. But if they feel bored and left out of life, they have every right to explain to her how they feel. They should discuss with her in what way they might contribute in a useful way to the activities of the household.

Older people have a great deal to contribute, and if they do so, they will integrate effectively with the rest of the family.

There is another factor which erodes good relationships. Self-pity is a characteristic which should be systematically and ruthlessly hounded out of our life. People who indulge in self-pity usually crave for warmth, affection and sympathy from those around them. But they cannot hope to attract such a response, for self-pity is, literally, a repellent trait.

Instead of voicing a grievance, voicing a wish is usually much more effective. For example, you may be lonely because your children do not visit you often enough. If you feel sorry for *yourself* you are likely to complain that they never make time to see you; this will make them feel guilty and resentful. More than likely they will not visit you any more frequently. But if you feel that you miss *their* company, and tell them so, your children will naturally feel pleased that they mean so much to you, and will be encouraged to see you more often.

A little forethought, planning, strategy and even cunning all have a place in shaping human relationships. They are not to be despised if they produce results which ensure a happier existence.

19

Individual Efforts and the Need for Social Reforms

As individuals we can do a great deal to keep ourselves from becoming frail and dependent – in other words a burden to ourselves, to our families and to society. We ourselves can ensure our health and well-being, but we need a supporting social and economic framework. Some of us are fortunate in having the inner resources and financial ease to be able to lead a varied and active life however old we are. Those less fortunately placed stand in especial need of certain measures which would help to make their post-retirement years worthwhile.

It is a fact that more people now live to be 70 and over, so that there are going to be increasing numbers of people who can contemplate the prospect of ten, fifteen, twenty or more years of retirement. What are all these people going to do with all these years? The whole of society will need to be involved in the solution to this question; otherwise, more and more of its resources will have to be spent on a growing population of ageing, unproductive and unwell citizens.

Life is organized in a rigid way at present: study or training; then work; then retirement at 60 or 65. After that follows free choice, which too often means no choice at all, but a 'drawing in of horns' and boredom. To be spending a quarter of one's life like this seems to make a mockery of all the earlier striving. Those of us who are either retired, or are nearing retirement – the senior citizens – are the ones who can agitate most effectively for rethinking and reform. Senior citizens are *voters*, and they have the right and the privilege to make their voices heard. A movement concerned with a better deal for the mature adult and for the older citizens would be a perfectly reasonable one. After all, *all of us* will, in due time, live many years as older citizens. It is self-evident that a better deal for the older citizens now means a better deal in old age for those who are young today. To mention but a few desirable reforms will illustrate some approaches to a better deal: more flexible retirement schedules, interchangeable pension and superannuation schemes, facilities for full-time or part-time study, extensive travel concessions, more opportunities for part-time employment without prejudice to pension rights, etc.

Whenever any new measure or reform is proposed the cost of its implementation is paramount. Too often the answer is that it will cost too much. So it would do, considered in isolation; but careful global costing may produce an entirely different picture. If senior citizens pressed for reforms they should not allow themselves to be fobbed off with a statement that to provide one facility or another 'will cost too much'. What is the *net cost* is the precise information required. After all, thousands of old people tucked away in geriatric wards, because they have nothing to live for, cost society a great deal in wasted resources and in cash. The extra cost of providing more elderly people with opportunities for remaining active may well be offset by an appreciable saving on geriatric and psychiatric hospital facilities. This is speaking brutally, solely in terms of cash. The savings in terms of human dignity and happiness are incalculable.

When more and more members of a society are in fact becoming senior citizens, that society needs to shape its institutions and policies in such a way as to provide for adults as a whole, not for specific age groups. Opportunities for employment or occupation, for study or for recreation, would then depend on a person's health, training, experience or interest, and *not* on their age. At present our obsessive quest for dates of birth and for specified age limits is quite ludicrous. Why should a post for an office typist be only suitable for someone aged 21–23?

Our names serve to identify us; our abilities and training serve to qualify us; our ages do neither.

20
Some Glimpses of Longevity

A short selection of long-lived people of renown
It is inspiriting to take a look at the life-span of prominent or renowned people through the ages. Some men of genius lived pathetically short lives, e.g. Mozart 35, Shelley 30, or Raphael 37. On the other hand, astonishing numbers of creative people lived, and live, to a very ripe old age: from the geometrician and philosopher Thales of Miletus, b. *circa* 636 BC (90), and the physician Hippocrates, b. *circa* 460 BC (104), to dramatist George Bernard Shaw, b. 1856 (94), and philosopher and mathematician Bertrand Russell, b. 1872 (98).

Such very long lived people represent a wide spectrum of activities. They include:

Composers: Heinrich Schütz, b. 1585 (87); Francesco Geminiani, b. 1667 (95); Gustave Charpentier, b. 1860 (96); Jan Sibelius, b. 1865 (92); Igor Stravinsky, b. 1882 (88).

Violin-makers: Four members of the Amati family, Antonio, b. 1550 (88), Girolamo I, b. 1551 (84), Nicolo, b. 1596 (88), and Girolamo II, b. 1649 (92); Antonio Stradivari, b. 1644 (93).

Executive musicians: Organist Johann Reinken, b. 1623 (99); violinist Giacomo Cervetto, b. 1682 (101); pianist Artur Rubinstein, b. 1885, living.

Architects: Giovanni Bernini, b. 1598 (82); Sir Christopher

Wren, b. 1632 (91); John Nash, b. 1752 (83); Frank Lloyd Wright, b. 1869 (90).

Sculptors: Donatello, b. 1382 (84); Luca della Robbia, b. 1399 (83); Michelangelo, b. 1475 (89).

Painters: Giovanni Bellini, b. 1422 (94); Lucas Cranach, b. 1472, (81); Titian, b. 1477 (99); Frans Hals, b. 1580 (86); Francisco Goya, b. 1746 (82); Katsushika Hokusai, b. 1760 (89); Edgar Degas, b. 1834 (83); Edvard Munch, b. 1863 (81); Pablo Picasso, b. 1881, living.

Poets: Anacreon, b. 570 BC (85); John Bellenden, b. 1495 (92); William Wordsworth, b. 1770 (80); Thomas Hardy, b. 1840 (88); Walter de la Mare, b. 1873 (83).

Novelists: H. G. Wells, b. 1866 (80); André Gide, b. 1869 (83); John Cowper Powys, b. 1872 (91); Somerset Maugham, b. 1874 (91); E. M. Forster, b. 1879 (91); Ivy Compton-Burnett, b. 1882 (87).

Dramatists: Sophocles, b. 495 BC (90); Metastasio, b. 1698 (84); Carlo Goldoni, b. 1707 (86); Maurice Maeterlinck, b. 1862 (87); Laurence Housman, b. 1865 (84).

Men-of-letters: Flavius Cassiodorus, b. 490 (93); Thomas Hobbes, b. 1588 (91); Calderon de la Barca, b. 1600 (81); Bernard de Fontenelle, b. 1657 (100); Voltaire, b. 1694 (84); Johann Wolfgang von Goethe, b. 1749 (83); Noah Webster, b. 1758 (85); John Ruskin, b. 1819 (81); Benedetto Croce, b. 1866 (86).

Philosophers: Diogenes, b. *circa* 412 BC (89); Saint Albertus Magnus, b. 1193 (107); Immanuel Kant, b. 1724 (80); Herbert Spencer, b. 1820 (83); Martin Buber, b. 1878 (87).

Natural philosophers: Democritus, b. *circa* 460 BC (90); Theophrastus, b. 370 BC (84); Roger Bacon, b. 1214 (80); Alexander von Humboldt, b. 1769 (90).

Scientists: Galileo Galilei, b. 1564 (78, executed); Anton van Leeuwenhoek, b. 1632 (91); Sir William Herschel, b. 1738 (84); Robert Bunsen, b. 1811 (88); Sir Joseph Hooker, b. 1817 (94); Jean Henri Fabre, b. 1825 (90); Sir Francis Galton, b. 1822 (89); Sir Clements Markham, b. 1830 (86); William Crookes, b. 1832 (87); Benjamin Emerson, b. 1843 (89); Ivan Pavlov, b. 1849 (87); Max Planck, b. 1858 (89); Sir Frederick Gowland Hopkins, b. 1861 (86).

Engineers, inventors: Otto von Guericke, b. 1602 (84); James Watt, b. 1736 (83); Sir Henry Bessemer, b. 1813 (85); John Fritz, b. 1823 (90); Alexandre Eiffel, b. 1832 (91); Thomas Alva Edison, b. 1847 (84); James Duryea, b. 1870 (97); Sir Barnes Wallis, b. 1887, living.

Physicians, psychologists: Galen, b. 129 (81); Gustav Fechner, b. 1801 (86); Sir Francis Haden, b. 1818 (92); Elizabeth Blackwell, b. 1821 (89); Joseph Lister, b. 1827 (85); Carl Jung, b. 1875 (86); Joseph Erlanger, b. 1877 (85).

Statesmen: Cato the Elder, b. 234 BC (86); Benjamin Franklin, b. 1706 (84); Thomas Jefferson, b. 1743 (83); William Gladstone, b. 1809 (89); Georges Clemenceau, b. 1841 (88); Jules Cambon, b. 1845 (90); Philippe Petain, b. 1856 (95); Mahatma Ghandi, b. 1869 (79, assassinated); Herbert Hoover, b. 1874 (90); Nancy Lady Astor, b. 1879 (85); Herbert Viscount Samuel, b. 1870 (93); Sir Winston Churchill, b. 1874 (91); Konrad Adenauer, b. 1876 (91); Harry S. Truman, b. 1884 (88).

Religious leaders: Gautama Buddha, b. 563 BC (80); Saint Anthony the Great, b. 251 (105); Pope Gregory IX, b. 1145 (96); John Wesley, b. 1703 (88); Cardinal John Henry Newman, b. 1801 (89); Mary Baker Eddy, b. 1821 (89); General William Booth, b. 1829 (83); Dean William Inge, b. 1860 (94); Pope John XXIII, b. 1881 (82); David McKay, b. 1874 (96).

Historians: Thomas Carlyle, b. 1795 (86); George Bancroft, b.

1800 (91); Cesare Cantu, b. 1804 (91); George Trevelyan, b. 1876 (86).

Educators: Philander Claxton, b. 1862 (95); Helen Keller, b. 1880 (87); Maria Montessori, b. 1870 (82).

Other activities not represented here are: rhetoricians, satirists, navigators, explorers, soldiers, sailors, jurists, political scientists, philanthropists, archaeologists, mathematicians, actors, economists, Egyptologists, women suffrage leaders, scene designers, musicologists, etc, etc. They similarly include many people of renown. The above long list of people represents no more than a small fraction of those found on a cursory search.

Creative capacity in old age

Even more inspiriting than mere longevity in famous people, is the realization how many of them continued to work with unabated verve and undiminished quality right up to their last days. Sophocles wrote his magnificent *Oedipus Coloneus* at 90. Death interrupted Plato (aged 87) in his task of writing the *Laws*. The Spartan General Agesilaus campaigned hard in the field, in person, at the age of 80. Titian was painting a 'Pieta' at the age of 99, when he died of the plague. Tintoretto was 72, when he completed the immense 'Paradise'. Michelangelo worked on the structure of St Peter's in Rome in his 80s. Thomas Mann, Leo Tolstoy, Victor Hugo and other writers produced important works in their 70s and 80s. In their 80s Giuseppe Verdi, Richard Strauss, Igor Stravinsky and Ralph Vaughan Williams composed some of their best music, in fact they were breaking new ground, seeking new modes of expression. Henri Matisse completed the decorations and the stained-glass windows for the Chapel at Vence in 1951, when aged 82. Finlay Currie was an actor for 70 years; Dame Sibyl Thorndike (b. 1882) is still acting today. The physiologist Pavlov was at the height of his powers at 86, when he died of pneumonia. Sir

Arthur Evans was still digging at Knossos in his 80s. Grandma Moses, the folk painter, took to painting when 78 and lived and painted to 101. The famous football coach Amos Stagg, after compulsory retirement (aged 70), refused to end his coaching career; his success thereafter was so outstanding that he was voted 'Coach of the Year' in 1943, when aged 81. He remained active and died aged 103.

Even handicaps did not curtail the activity of some. In the last years of his life Auguste Renoir, then in his 70s, could paint only with brushes strapped to his hands, but produced masterpieces. Although handicapped by cataracts before he was 60, Claude Monet painted huge canvasses into his 80s, using a bolder technique. Mercator, the geographer, at 80 wrote a treatise, when half-paralysed by a stroke.

Conductors

It seems that orchestral conductors have a special place among those whose quality improves as they grow older. In fact on present form it would seem that the 'peak' of a great conductor's work is between 70 and 90. The habitual physical exertion of a conductor's life, coupled with dedication to his art, and a role which shapes the efforts of others, must be a very fortunate combination of factors. In recent memory great octogenarian conductors have included: Arturo Toscanini, Pierre Monteux, Tullio Serafin, Sir Thomas Beecham, Leopold Stokowski, Bruno Walter, Otto Klemperer, Ernest Ansermet, Vittorio Gui, Carl Schuricht.

Our ideas about longevity

Taking a look at the creative cream of the population makes one realize, that, although they represent an élite, they must also reflect something of the general human condition. There must be many more vital old people than any of us imagine. We know nothing about them, because they are ordinary people.

In 1850 2.5 per cent of the population of the U.S.A. were 65 or over; by 1970 this proportion had increased to 10 per cent. Thus about 20 million Americans are over 65!

If you are told that of 100 people today aged 50, 99 are likely to be alive in a year's time, and you are then asked to hazard a guess as to how many of 100 people today aged 80 will still be alive next year, what would you say – 40, 50 or even 60? In fact, of the 100 80-year olds 89 will become 81! Even at 90 years 77 per cent are likely to reach their 91st birthday!

Index

Ageing (pathological) 28
Ageing (physiological) 28
Alcoholic drinks 91
Anabolic steroids 97
Anaemia 96
Animal fats 23
Apathy 61
Atherosclerosis 23, 88
Attitudes to ageing 62

Biological élite 22
Body image 48

Calcium 96
Calendar age 55, 60, 67, 69
Cataracts 83
Challenges 37
Contact with other age groups 66, 118
Coronaries 89
Creative capacity in old age 127

Deafness 83
Depression 78, 81
Dietary habits 90

Effort 53
Environment 23, 31
Exercises (daily) 106
Eye-sight 82, 83

Family relationships 119
Fear of old age 38
Feet 84, 85
Fluids 91

Gardening 54, 101
Glaucoma 83
Golf 55, 102

Health criteria 80
Health surveillance clinics 79
Hearing 82, 83, 84
Heredity and longevity 21, 126
Holidays 103

Image of old age 31
Interdependence of mental and physical
    factors 116
Iron 96
Isolation 67

Kinesophilia 76

Life as a continuum 59
Life-span 21
Longevity 21, 36, 124, 128

Malnutrition 87
Medical check-ups 77
Medicines 97, 114
'Mental arthritis' 64, 65, 118
Mental decline 28
Mental flexibility 65
Mental stimulation 117
Metabolic processes 17
Milestones 59, 60
Minerals 96
Mobility (general) 98
Movement 47

'Norms' 60
Nutrition 86

Obesity 86
'Old age' 34
'Opting out' 63, 67
Osteoporosis 96
'Out of condition' 49

Participation 61
Peak of performance 69
Performance 55, 69
Phobias 78
Physical activity 46, 49
Physical capacity 53
Physical decline 27
Positive health 75, 77
Positive philosophy of ageing 60
Potential in old age 25, 43
Prime (of life) 33

Recreation 71
Rejuvenation 12
Relaxation 117
Research into ageing 30
Rest 19, 50, 53
Restoration 53

Retirement 61, 121

Safety measures 111
Self-pity 120
Senility 24
Smoking 92
Sports 102
Stairs climbing 99, 101, 111
Standards of performance 71
Strokes 89
Swimming 36, 55, 102

Table-tennis 102
Taking it easy 18
Training 55, 103

Undernutrition 88

Values 62
View of life (dynamic) 16
View of life (mechanistic) 16, 18
Visits to the doctor 78
Vitality 11, 37
Vitamin C 90
Vitamins 93

Walking 100
Wear and tear 16